EPIDURAL WITHOUT GUILT

Childbirth Without Pain

EPIDURAL WITHOUT GUILT

Childbirth Without Pain

Gilbert J. Grant, MD

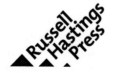

White Plains, New York
www.russellhastingspress.com

Epidural Without Guilt: Childbirth Without Pain

Copyright © 2011 by Gilbert J. Grant, MD

Manufactured in the United States of America

All rights reserved

Published by Russell Hastings Press, Ltd.

P.O. Box 229, White Plains, New York 10605

Russell Hastings Press books may be purchased for educational, business, or promotional use. For information, contact Russell Hastings Press, Ltd. in writing at P.O. Box 229, White Plains, NY 10605 or by e mail at sales@RussellHastingsPress.com.

First edition, First printing

ISBN 978-0-9759939-3-4

Library of Congress Control Number: 2010903230

Cover Design by Bookwrights

Cartoon Illustrations by David Zinn

Medical Illustrations by P. Jasmine Katatikarn

Visit: www.EpiduralWithoutGuilt.com
for educational video animations and additional information.

BEFORE YOU BEGIN READING...

CONTENTS

ACKNOWLEDGMENTS

It is difficult to imagine having completed this book without the sage advice, guidance, and hard work of my father and my teacher, Dr. Abraham H. Grant. His tireless assistance and input at every stage of writing and production cannot be overstated. But his role in molding my character has been more important. As exhibited through his instruction, and even more so by his example, my father's genuine concern for his patients indelibly shaped my approach to relieving the suffering of women in labor.

How fortunate I am to have been influenced by a wonderful human being and great clinician, Dr. Sivam Ramanathan, my instructor and mentor in obstetric anesthesia and dear friend for more than a quarter-century. I am also indebted to my beloved late brother-in-law, Dr. Ken Weissman, a gifted obstetrician who profoundly influenced my career choice.

The impetus to write *Epidural Without Guilt* came from the many women for whom I have been privileged to care. But its publication would not have been possible without the great understanding and considerable patience of my wife, Judy, and our daughters, Alexandra, Tori, and Sydney. Their loving encouragement is a constant source of strength.

Gilbert J. Grant, MD
New York, NY

PREFACE

Why I Wrote This Book
and
Why You Should Read It

As an anesthesiologist, I have been caring for women during childbirth for twenty-five years. I specialize in relieving the pain of labor and delivery using the most effective and reliable means available: epidurals and/or spinals. The most frustrating aspect of my job is watching fear, guilt, and misinformation make up women's minds on childbirth pain relief before they've had a chance to do so for themselves.

Many mothers-to-be are quite concerned about the safety of labor pain relief techniques. The thought of receiving an epidural, which involves inserting a needle into the lower back, can be unsettling. And mere mention of the term "spinal" can heighten the dread, compounded by frightening stories women may have heard about anesthesia. So this double-edged fear—of labor pain itself and of the techniques used to treat it—can cause anxiety for months before delivery.

In addition, women attending childbirth education classes, predominantly first-time mothers-to-be, often report that instructors put a negative spin on epidurals and spinals, dismissing them as "unnatural" or even harmful interventions. If some women worry that their request for labor pain relief will be interpreted as a sign of weakness, others fear it will harm their baby, a fallacy you will come to understand after reading this book.

During my wife's first pregnancy, back in 1993, I browsed through the materials she was reading and found that although many of them discussed a variety of ways to manage the pain of childbirth, none presented the full picture of epidurals/spinals, even though these techniques are used by nearly three in four of women who give birth in the United States. Worse still, the information presented was often incorrect.

So in 1996, to better inform and educate patients about epidurals and spinals, I began offering a monthly seminar at New York University Langone Medical Center, where I work and teach. The success of this program persuaded me to extend its reach by writing *Enjoy Your Labor*, published in 2005.

Based on the questions expectant mothers have asked me over the years, *Enjoy Your Labor* was designed to demystify epidural/spinal techniques by detailing what to expect in easy-to-understand terms. I find that once women have a thorough understanding of what's involved, they are much less anxious about receiving pain relief, and perhaps about the process of delivery itself.

Another key point I sought to convey—and one not emphasized in any book I came across—was the advantage of getting epidurals/spinals early in the course of labor. My philosophy is common sense: If you choose to have the best pain relief possible for labor and delivery, get it before severe pain begins. All too frequently, women receive their epidural after labor pain becomes unbearable, the way childbirth pain traditionally has been handled.

To foster informed decision-making about childbirth pain relief, it was also critical to debunk the many myths surrounding epidurals/ spinals. Without doubt, these misconceptions color the ability to judge whether labor pain relief is right for you. Five years later, however, I am disheartened to report that myths regarding pain relief for childbirth remain entrenched and continue to be communicated in subtle and not-so-subtle ways.

Recently, a woman whose epidural turned agony into a comfortable birth experience told me afterward that her yoga teacher had warned the class about the dangers of epidurals. This new mother lamented that other students may have been dissuaded from taking advantage of what she discovered was a very good thing indeed.

Also, since *Enjoy Your Labor* was published, more research has come to light that shows a connection between unrelieved pain during and immediately after childbirth and the development of serious long-term problems for mother and child. These problems include psychiatric disorders such as post-partum depression and post-traumatic stress disorder, as well as chronic pain.

To inform expectant mothers about these important new findings, and debunk the still-present myths surrounding epidurals/spinals, I decided to write *Epidural Without Guilt*. As you will learn from reading this book, rather than harming you or your baby, an epidural/spinal can actually benefit you both. But since most women—and men—are not aware of this, needless trepidation continues to inject an unhealthy dose of guilt into pain relief decision-making.

This new edition was also fueled by the women who told me they found *Enjoy Your Labor* informative, that it helped them to cope with some of the uncertainties of childbirth. Like them, you will see the logic behind getting an epidural as soon as it is clear you are truly in labor, and before the pain becomes severe. You'll learn the benefits of relieving pain not only during labor, but also after delivery, during the postpartum period. And you'll come to understand that you should feel no guilt about choosing the best type of pain relief available.

This book is written from my perspective as an obstetric anesthesiologist practicing in a major teaching hospital where medical advances are introduced, and where my colleagues and I provide full-time coverage in the labor and delivery suite. At smaller facilities, anesthesiologists may serve obstetric patients on an as-needed basis, so certain techniques I describe may not be available. Learn which options you will have long before labor commences.

A clear understanding of the process of labor pain relief will reduce fear about your upcoming delivery. Empower yourself with knowledge so you can make an informed choice. Knowing what to expect in terms of pain management will help to focus your thoughts on the one that is most important: joyful anticipation of your new baby.

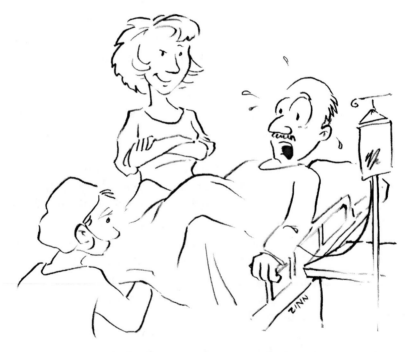

A sure way for women to experience painless childbirth

1

WHY IS CHILDBIRTH PAIN VIEWED DIFFERENTLY FROM ALL OTHER TYPES OF PAIN?

 ## Topics to Be Delivered

- Is a double standard in effect for women giving birth?
- Is "natural" always better?
- The role of guilt in childbirth pain relief
- Every woman should decide for herself whether she wants pain relief

Imagine this: you are being wheeled in to have your appendix removed when a member of the surgical team peers down from above his mask and says, "Tell you what we'll do. Bear up as best you can without anesthesia, and if it gets too rough we'll give you something for the pain." Sounds crazy, right? No man would be asked to submit to an appendectomy, which can be performed in twenty-four minutes, without anesthesia. Yet the severe pain of labor, which can persist for more than twenty-four hours, is somehow viewed as a condition women should simply endure, since childbirth is a natural process—as if "natural" pain is any less intense than that induced by a surgeon's scalpel. In fact, the pain of childbirth is the worst pain most women will experience in a lifetime.

So why is there so much prejudice against epidurals and spinals? Part of the explanation is that women are often treated as second-class citizens. How else can one explain why pain relief for labor is still considered an option or a luxury? Menstrual cramps, which pale in comparison to labor contractions, are routinely treated with pain relievers. Why does anyone question whether labor pain merits treatment? As more than a few women have observed, if men had labor pain, its relief would probably be viewed quite differently.

SYMPATHY PAIN

The Huichol Indians of north-central Mexico sought to make childbirth a more equitable experience. Their interesting birthing practice, illustrated in fig. 1-1, intimately involved the father-to-be in the process.

"According to Huichol tradition, when a woman had her first child, the husband squatted in the rafters of the house, or in the branches of a tree, directly above her, with ropes attached to his scrotum. As she went into labor pain, the wife pulled vigorously on the ropes, so that her husband shared in the painful, but ultimately joyous, experience of childbirth."[1]

It's difficult to imagine that methodology going over big with even the most sympathetic men in the United States. Instead, on the other end of the spectrum exists a school of thought that epidurals/spinals will deprive the mother of the ecstasy of giving birth, literally. Orgasmic Birth adherents believe that with proper preparation, the moment of birth will be accompanied by an intense climax that will not be experienced if a woman uses an epidural/spinal—yet another reason to avoid state-of-the-art pain relief. You just can't make this stuff up!

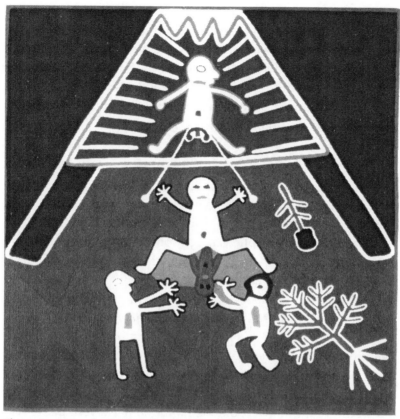

Fig. 1-1. *How the husband assists in the birth of a child. The tradition of the Huichol Indians of north-central Mexico. Reproduced with permission of the Fine Arts Museums of San Francisco.*

THE NO PAIN, NO GAIN MYTH

Strange thing about the pain of labor and delivery: many women are taught to believe they should simply tolerate it or "tough it out," that all good things require some sacrifice. The message is that the joy of childbirth is much more profound when preceded by the bearing of pain.

Although many natural childbirth folks ascribe to this philosophy, a healthy percentage of people do not view labor through a "no pain, no gain" prism. I recently cared for a woman who competes in Ironman contests, which comprise swimming,

7

cycling, and running marathons. She told me that the rigors of these competitions, while severe, did not compare to labor, the worst pain this Ironwoman had ever experienced. She hired a doula to help her deal with her labor, but after ten hours, the elite athlete saw no reason to endure what she judged to be a no-win situation. She requested an epidural and an hour later delivered a beautiful baby boy.

NATURAL WOMAN

The term "natural" implies that a birth in which the mother receives pain medication is somehow unnatural. (Who would ever choose "unnatural" childbirth?) Unnatural sounds plain silly, though, when applied to, say, pneumonia, for which you can take penicillin or do it the natural way and die. Granted, these two conditions are inherently different: unlike untreated disease, the pain of labor and delivery will not kill anyone. But I attach no less importance to its treatment.

I vividly recall a conversation with a physician who told me that once he informs laboring women that the pain they are experiencing is a natural part of childbirth, it becomes bearable. Interesting, I thought. If someone told me the severe pain I was experiencing was natural, I do not think it would hurt any less: I would want relief, and quickly!

Pregnant Pause

"Natural" pain may hurt just as much or even more than "unnatural" pain. Both can be treated—if that's what you want.

"Natural childbirth" preparation can also be a setup for feeling inadequate. Some childbirth educators teach that if you learn breathing and focusing techniques and practice them properly, you'll be able to avoid pain medication. But for many mothers-to-be, this approach is doomed to fail when breathing and focusing do not adequately mitigate their pain. When the woman in labor uses the techniques she's been coached in but still experiences unbearable pain, she may think it's all her fault: "If only I had paid more attention in class and learned how to do the breathing better, it wouldn't hurt now." If she ends up asking for and receiving an epidural, she may feel like even more of a failure.

Epidural Episodes:
BIRTH PANGS AND PANGS OF CONSCIENCE

F.S. was a first-time mother-to-be who was convinced she did not want any type of pain medication for labor. She was highly motivated and had dutifully attended a childbirth education course that instructed her in breathing and focusing techniques that would eliminate the need for anesthesia. But as her labor pains became more intense and far more severe than she had imagined, breathing and focusing proved no match for the pain. Still, she was determined to avoid an epidural. After six agonizing hours, she finally tired of her pain and begged for an epidural. We immediately gave her one, which worked as intended, relieving all her pain within fifteen minutes. I thought she would be pleased, now that her agony had ended. But when I visited her room a half-hour later she was crying uncontrollably—out of guilt for having taken the epidural. What a scene: completely comfortable, no longer feeling her contractions, she thought she had failed some kind of test. This dramatically demonstrates the problem with "natural" approaches: a woman is made to feel like a failure if she asks for pain relief.

EASY WAY OUT?

That mothers-to-be are made to feel guilty for requesting pain relief is especially unfortunate considering what state-of-the-art obstetric anesthesia techniques can offer. Their stigmatization as an "easy way out" that compromises the safety of both mother and child is nonsense, of course, but many women buy into this faulty reasoning.

9

Not only are today's epidurals/spinals safe for the overwhelming majority of mothers and babies, they have also been demonstrated to deliver beneficial long-term effects. And while the problems that can occur with childbirth anesthesia are broadly discussed, what's largely unnoted are short- and long-term risks posed by not choosing an epidural/spinal. Chapters 9 and 10 will bring you up to speed on these.

Pregnant Pause
Consider your options for pain relief carefully before labor begins. When you are in the throes of labor pain, you will not be in the best condition to weigh these options objectively.

ONLY YOU CAN JUDGE

Pain is a completely subjective sensation; no one else can judge how much or how little you are experiencing. Individuals not in labor (doctors, midwives, nurses, and coaches) tend to underestimate the intensity of the woman's suffering; yet these are the people who often advise on whether it should be alleviated.

Physicians who treat labor pain, meanwhile, are quite clear on the subject. In the words of the Australian anesthesiologist Dr. Peter Brownridge, "To pretend that natural childbirth is other than very painful for most women can only be described as a cruel and callous deception."[2] It should be your call, so make sure it is: learn what to expect during labor and delivery and find out what options are available, so you can make an informed decision about what pain relief, if any, you want.

Key Concepts to Carry Away
Although many women are made to feel guilty for wanting childbirth pain relief, approximately three in four end up requesting and receiving an epidural/spinal. Don't let anyone else make the decision for you. Empower yourself by obtaining the knowledge you need to choose which technique will be best when you deliver your baby.

2

CAUSES OF CHILDBIRTH PAIN AND STRATEGIES FOR ITS RELIEF

Topics to Be Delivered

- **The origins of pain during the different stages of labor and delivery**
- **Two different approaches to pain relief: Systemic versus regional**
- **Why regional pain relief is the most effective option for childbirth**

THE BASIS FOR PAIN

What is the cause of pain? Why does something hurt? Pain begins when a part of the body is cut, stretched, pressed, or exposed to heat or extreme cold. This starts a pain message that travels through the nerves—the body's communication system—first to the spinal cord and then up to the brain. When the message arrives in the brain we perceive the pain. This entire process happens in less than a second.

THE STAGES OF LABOR AND PERCEPTION OF PAIN

As labor progresses, the pain message originates from different locations. Labor is divided into three stages. It begins with the onset of regular uterine contractions, which cause the cervix, the outlet at the base of the uterus through which the baby passes into the vagina, to open, or dilate. The first stage of labor ends when the cervix is fully dilated, to a diameter of ten centimeters.

Pain during the first stage is caused by contractions of the uterus and stretching of the cervix. At the beginning of labor, the contractions produce a sensation that is at first uncomfortable, often likened to bad menstrual cramps, but which gradually becomes more intense. Women perceive first-stage pains in different locations, most commonly in the lower abdomen, but many also feel them in their back. Some also feel the pain in their buttocks, hips, and thighs.

When the cervix is dilated to about seven or eight centimeters the pain becomes even more intense. During this interval, known as "transition" (from first to second stage), some women experience nausea and vomiting. During the second stage, as the baby descends through the birth canal, pain is caused in two ways: by the contracting uterus and also by the stretching and sometimes tearing of tissue in the cervix, vagina, and perineum, the area between the vagina and anus.

The second stage of labor, also known as the pushing stage, ends with delivery of the baby. The third stage is the interval between the birth of the baby and delivery of the placenta.

WHEN WILL LABOR PAIN START AND HOW SEVERE WILL IT BE?

Because each woman has a unique experience with labor pain, it is not possible to predict accurately what she will feel. Furthermore, the same woman may have a very different pain experience from one labor to the next. Some women have more pain earlier in labor; a very few do not experience much pain at all. In general, the pain of early contractions is less severe than the pain that occurs later as labor progresses.

The intensity and location of the pain may also depend on the baby's position as it descends through the birth canal. For example, if the baby's head is positioned to emerge face-up, the mother is more likely to have pain in the lower back ("back labor").

Pregnant Pause

For most women, childbirth is the worst pain that they will ever experience—but for those choosing epidurals and/or spinals, the pain can be prevented.

SYSTEMIC VERSUS REGIONAL PAIN RELIEF

Two approaches are used to treat the pain of childbirth with medication: systemic and regional. With the systemic approach, medication is given throughout the entire body, or system, and a portion makes its way to the brain, where it blunts the perception of pain. With the regional approach, a relatively small dose of medication is administered into the epidural or spinal space, to block the pain message from being transmitted to the brain.

The systemic drugs most commonly used in labor are the narcotics Demerol, morphine, Stadol, and Nubain. They are injected into a vein or a muscle and they exert their effects in the brain to diminish perception of pain. Because little technical expertise is required to administer systemic medication, their use does not require the presence of an anesthesiologist; so if an anesthesiologist is not available, the systemic approach makes sense. It has many disadvantages, however. Patients tend to feel drowsy after receiving systemically administered narcotics. Nausea and vomiting often occur. Furthermore, because a relatively large dose is used, a considerable amount of the drug may be transferred to the baby, making the newborn sleepy and slowing his or her breathing.

But the main downside of systemic narcotics is that they do not relieve labor pain effectively. They often cause the mother-to-be to fall asleep between contractions, only to have her wake up groaning in pain during contractions.

Once it is established that a woman is truly in labor, there is no reason to use systemic narcotics unless she is not able to receive an epidural or a spinal for one of the specific medical reasons listed in chapter 7.

Because regional pain relief—again, fundamentally different in that it stops pain before it reaches the brain—is administered directly into the epidural or spinal space, much smaller doses of medication are required. One result is fewer side effects. The mother's state of mind is not altered, and very little medication reaches the baby. Additional benefits and aspects of spinal/ epidural techniques are described in the following chapter.

Key Concepts to Carry Away

Regional pain relief techniques—epidurals and spinals—are based on the administration of small doses of anesthetics very close to the location of the nerves that carry the pain message. Unlike systemic techniques, regional techniques keep the mother-to-be pain free and clear-headed. If labor pain is severe enough to warrant treatment, why not choose the most effective means available to get maximal pain relief with a minimum of side effects for you and your baby?

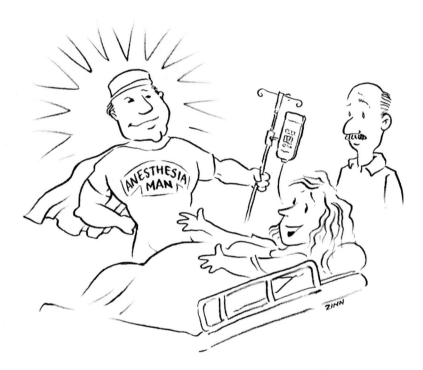

"Where have you been all my life?"

3

FROM BETTER TO BEST: CHILDBIRTH PAIN RELIEF THEN AND NOW

Topics to Be Delivered

- Who was the first American to have anesthesia during childbirth?
- Royal pain and the development of obstetric anesthesia
- What did your mother and grandmother have for pain relief?
- What is an epidural?
- What is a spinal?
- The role of the modern anesthesiologist in relieving the pain of labor and delivery

Pain relief for childbirth followed the introduction of ether and chloroform anesthesia for general surgery in 1846. The surgical patient would inhale these anesthetic gases into the lungs, and then fall into an unconscious state. Within a few months of introducing anesthetic gases in surgical practice, physicians began to use them to relieve the pain of labor and delivery. The dream of pain-free childbirth was on its way to becoming a reality.

On January 19, 1847, the renowned Scottish obstetrician Dr. James Young Simpson administered ether to relieve labor pain. Four months later in the United States, Dr. Nathan Cooley Keep, a Massachusetts dentist and physician, gave ether to Fanny Appleton Longfellow, the wife of the poet Henry Wadsworth Longfellow, for the birth of their third child. Having experienced two previous deliveries without the benefit of pain relief, Fanny Longfellow was well qualified to speak on the subject. She extolled the virtues of anesthesia as "certainly the greatest blessing of this age."[3]

Six years later, Queen Victoria's physician, Dr. John Snow, anesthetized her with chloroform to ease the pain of delivering her seventh child, Prince Leopold. When her eldest daughter gave birth in 1860, the Queen remarked, "What a blessing she had chloroform!"— a clarion call for its popularization and the title of Dr. Donald Caton's 1999 history of the subject.[4]

As Caton notes, on both sides of the Atlantic, the concept was opposed as strongly as it was embraced. Some leading obstetricians of the day viewed the use of anesthesia in childbirth as interference with the natural order of things. "The pain of labor had never been great enough to prevent women from having more children," said the mid-nineteenth century Philadelphia-based obstetrician Dr. Charles D. Meigs.

Physicians like Meigs argued that systemic anesthetics would harm the uterus and the progress of labor, and that inducing unconsciousness could be unsafe for the mother. There was also concern that anesthetic gases administered to the mother would cross the placenta and have detrimental effects on the newborn, making the baby sleepy and sluggish, and possibly subject to other, unknown long-term side effects.

Others were opposed to childbirth pain relief on philosophical or religious grounds. Some physicians based their argument on an edict from Genesis 3:16, "In pain shall you bear children"— Eve's punishment for tempting Adam with the forbidden fruit.

Social attitudes toward pain in general were quite complex, but during the nineteenth century they underwent tremendous change. Physicians who became adept at administering the new anesthetics witnessed dramatic results in their patients, and their experience transformed them into passionate proponents of the methodology. Their enthusiasm for the comfort they were able to provide outweighed the risk of any side effects they may have observed.

The enlightened public began to praise the ability of doctors to alleviate pain: they viewed it as a human triumph over the dark forces of nature. This philosophical view, widely held in Europe and America at the time, provided a receptive audience for the argument favoring anesthesia in childbirth. Ultimately, it gained widespread acceptance because women themselves insisted that their physicians provide pain relief.

Negative attitudes that persist today are based more on "scientific" considerations than religious ones. For example, some argue that the potential harm to baby, mother, or the progress of labor outweighs the benefits. Natural childbirth enthusiasts say pain relievers may lead to a cascade of other interventions requiring the use of forceps or even a cesarean delivery, concerns I discuss in chapter 11.

TWILIGHT SLEEP

In 1903, an alternative to ether and chloroform for relief of childbirth pain was introduced in Europe. The new systemic technique was the injection of a narcotic, morphine, combined with the drug scopolamine to create a state called "twilight sleep." In this condition, the mother had no recollection of the pain of delivery, owing to the potent amnesia-producing properties of scopolamine.

Twilight sleep's prime advantage was the relative simplicity of the procedure: it was much easier to give a patient an injection than to have her inhale an anesthetic gas. But twilight sleep proved to be less than ideal for childbirth. Morphine did not relieve pain completely, while scopolamine prevented the woman from remembering the extraordinary act of giving birth. The result was an incoherent mother with no memory of the delivery. Moreover, morphine resulted in sleepy newborns: some had significant problems breathing, while others were born asphyxiated. Despite these drawbacks, twilight sleep was very popular, and some women in the United States continued to use it as late as the 1960s.

Pregnant Pause

With twilight sleep, women were unaware of their delivery. We now know that this wasn't such a great idea. Not only did mothers miss the exciting moment of birth, but being essentially unconscious exposed them and their babies to serious medical risks as well.

DEMEROL AND OTHER NARCOTICS

Another injectable systemic narcotic, Demerol, was introduced in labor and delivery suites in the United States in 1948. Like morphine, Demerol produces more drowsiness than pain relief and is associated with many side effects, including nausea, vomiting, and itching. It may also cause a slow rate of breathing in the newborn. Despite these drawbacks, Demerol achieved immense popularity, and it is still used in many hospitals.

Other injectable narcotic medications have also been used over the years to treat labor pain. Stadol, preferred by some over Demerol because it is less likely to slow breathing, occasionally causes feelings of anxiety, depression, restlessness, and/or hallucinations. Other narcotics used include Nubain, fentanyl, sufentanil, and remifentanil.

In addition to the drowsiness, nausea, vomiting, and itching a systemic narcotic can cause in mothers-to-be, its administration can make the fetal heart rate monitor difficult to interpret. As mentioned above, systemic narcotics may also cause problems after delivery by slowing down the breathing rate in the newborn.

At one minute after birth babies whose mothers received systemic narcotics have lower Apgar scores—a general measure of neonatal well-being—and a greater likelihood of requiring additional medication (Narcan) to reverse the effects of the narcotics than babies of mothers who received epidurals. Remifentanil, because it is the shortest-acting narcotic, has the advantage of not causing breathing problems in the newborn, but it is more complicated to administer, requires more intensive monitoring of the mother, and is not yet available everywhere.

Nowadays, the best way to administer narcotics is with an intravenous patient controlled analgesia (PCA) system. PCA lets you push a button connected to an electronic pump that triggers a narcotic injection directly into your vein. The pump is programmed so that you cannot overdose yourself.

For women who cannot or do not want to have an epidural or spinal, intravenous PCA is the next-best choice. For labor pain relief, the most popular narcotics used with intravenous PCA are fentanyl and remifentanil. Intravenous PCA is also used to provide pain relief after delivery (chapter 8).

Pregnant Pause

Narcotics such as Demerol and morphine administered systemically during labor are not very effective pain relievers and may cause many side effects in the mother-to-be such as drowsiness, nausea and vomiting, and slowing of breathing.

REGIONAL PAIN RELIEF

Local or regional anesthetics, which block the pain message from traveling through nerves, were first used for general surgery in the 1880s. Not long afterward scientists discovered that injection of local anesthetic into the epidural or spinal space within the vertebral column produced profound relief of pain. (The anatomical name of the spaces are used to describe the procedures, hence the common use of the terms "epidural" or "spinal" to refer to these techniques of pain relief.) By the mid-twentieth century, epidurals/spinals were being used in the labor room, so women were able to have their pain relieved yet remain awake and alert to fully experience the delivery of their baby.

EPIDURALS

The epidural space is located in the spinal column just outside the dura, a layer of tissue that surrounds the spinal fluid (figure 3-1). The epidural space can be reached using different approaches. From the 1930s through the 1960s, anesthesiologists commonly performed epidurals by inserting a needle through the caudal portion of the vertebral column, which is located very low in the back, just above the coccyx (tailbone).This procedure became known as a "caudal." By the 1970s the caudal was replaced by the lumbar approach, in which the needle is placed higher up in the back (figure 3-2). Today, nearly all labor epidurals are placed using the lumbar approach.

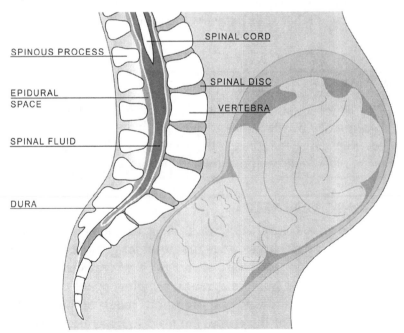

Fig. 3-1. *Side view (cross-section) of the abdomen and lower back.*

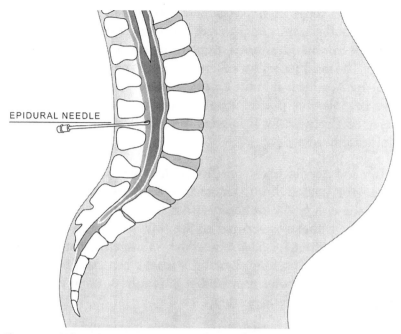

EPIDURAL NEEDLE

Fig. 3-2. *Side view (cross-section) of the lower portion of the vertebral column showing the epidural needle, with its tip in the epidural space.*

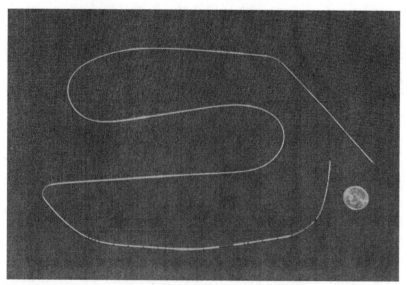

Fig. 3-3. *Epidural catheter. The dime is shown for size comparison. Only three to four inches of the end of the catheter are inserted through the epidural needle into the back.*

Once the needle tip is positioned within the epidural space, a local anesthetic may be injected. But a single dose lasts for only twenty to ninety minutes, depending on which anesthetic is used. The need for repeated needle insertions can be avoided by placing a catheter into the epidural space. An epidural catheter is a tiny flexible plastic tube through which the anesthetic is injected (figure 3-3). It is very thin, so it can fit through the epidural needle.

After the needle tip is positioned in the epidural space, the catheter is passed through it, and the needle is removed, leaving only the end of the catheter within the epidural space (figure 3-4). The catheter is secured to the skin with adhesive tape. It can remain there for days, if need be—although labor hopefully does not last that long. Local anesthetic can then be injected through the catheter repeatedly as required, to provide pain relief for as long as is needed.

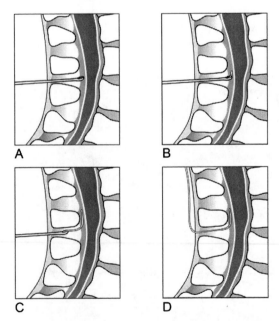

Fig. 3-4. *Insertion of an epidural catheter. A: The tip of the epidural needle is positioned within the epidural space. B: The epidural catheter is threaded through the epidural needle into the epidural space. C: The epidural needle being removed. D: The epidural needle is completely removed, leaving only the epidural catheter within the epidural space.*

TECHNOLOGICAL ADVANCES

During the 1980s, anesthesiologists began using electronic pumps to administer local anesthetic continuously in order to maintain pain relief. Widely adopted during the 1990s, this practice was a great improvement because it provided a constant level of comfort instead of the peaks and valleys of pain and relief that had been the rule with intermittent dosing. The epidural catheter is hooked up to a pump attached to a pole on wheels, the same pole on which an intravenous infusion bag is hung, allowing the woman to walk around during labor if she so desires (figure 3-5).

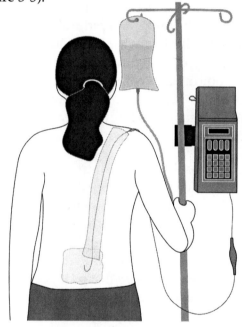

Fig. 3-5. *Epidural catheter taped to the back and connected to an infusion pump. The pump is attached to a pole on wheels—the same one on which the i.v. fluid bag hangs—allowing the woman to walk if she desires.*

An anesthesiologist practicing thirty years ago would hardly recognize the "walking epidural" used today. The earliest epidurals produced profound muscle weakness in the legs, immobilizing the mother-to-be below the waist. For today's walking epidural, relatively dilute local anesthetics are used. These low-dose anesthetics cause less muscle weakness, so the woman can walk during labor if she desires and is able to push the baby out more effectively when the time comes.

Another advancement is that since the early days of epidurals, new and better local anesthetics have been discovered. Also, small doses of other types of pain relievers that do not produce muscle weakness, such as synthetic narcotics, are now administered together with the local anesthetics. The result is excellent pain relief with minimal effects on muscle strength.

SPINALS

A "spinal" refers to the injection of pain-relieving medication into the spinal fluid. Unlike an epidural, the spinal needle is passed through the dura into the spinal fluid, and a single dose of medication is injected (figure 3-6). Spinals take effect more quickly than epidurals—within three to five minutes as compared to ten to fifteen minutes—but don't last as long. Spinal pain relief wears off within a few hours, in contrast with the days of pain relief possible with an epidural catheter.

Before 1987, spinals had fallen into disfavor for childbirth because as many as 20 percent of women suffered a severe, incapacitating headache that necessitated many days' bed rest after delivery. The problem—symptoms and treatment of which are described in chapter 9—is caused by leakage of spinal fluid through the hole made in the dura. But the "pencil-point" needle tip, a major innovation in design that produces a different shape of hole in the dura, dramatically reduced the incidence of post-spinal headache to only 1 to 2 percent of patients, making the spinal route a reasonable option for childbirth pain relief.

Pregnant Pause

One difference between a spinal and an epidural is the location where the medication is injected. With an epidural, it is injected into the epidural space, outside of the dura. With a spinal, it is injected slightly deeper (about one-quarter of an inch), through the dura and into the spinal fluid.

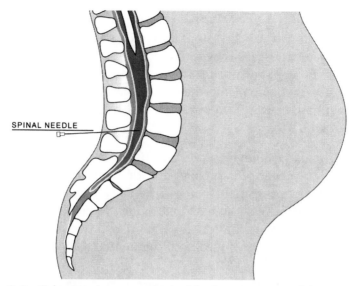

SPINAL NEEDLE

Fig. 3-6. *Side view (cross-section) of the lower portion of the vertebral column showing the spinal needle, with its tip passed through the dura into the spinal space.*

COMBINED SPINAL-EPIDURAL

Today, spinals and epidurals are often used interchangeably; in fact, they are sometimes used together. With a combined spinal-epidural, the epidural needle is first inserted into the epidural space. Next, a spinal needle is passed through the epidural needle.

Because the spinal needle used for this technique is longer than the epidural needle, the tip of the spinal needle extends past the tip of the epidural needle, pierces the dura, and comes to rest within the spinal fluid. Anesthetic is then injected into the spinal fluid and the spinal needle is withdrawn. Next, an epidural catheter is threaded through the epidural needle, and the epidural needle is removed, leaving only the epidural catheter in place (figure 3-7).

The reasons for choosing an epidural, a spinal, or a combined spinal-epidural are delineated in chapter 4. And you can view video animations of the epidural and spinal procedures at www.EpiduralWithoutGuilt.com.

THE MODERN ANESTHESIOLOGIST

When anesthesia was first used for childbirth 150 years ago, the specialty of anesthesiology did not yet exist. At that time, anesthetics were administered by obstetricians, dentists, and others. The specialty of anesthesiology was not established until the twentieth century, when residency training programs were developed.

Today's anesthesiologist attends four years of medical school, followed by a year of internship and three more years' specialized training as a resident in anesthesiology. Our primary job in the labor and delivery suite is to provide pain relief, but we are also trained in resuscitation. So even if you decide against an epidural/spinal, you can feel confident with an anesthesiologist nearby.

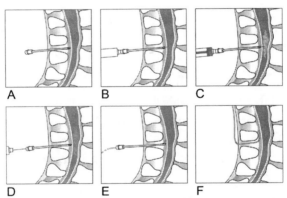

Fig. 3-7. *Combined spinal-epidural. A: Epidural needle with its tip in the epidural space. B: Spinal needle passed through epidural needle and through dura so that its tip rests within the spinal fluid. C: medication injected into the spinal fluid. D: spinal needle being removed. E: Epidural catheter passed through epidural needle into epidural space. F: The epidural needle has been completely removed leaving only the epidural catheter within the epidural space.*

Key Concepts to Carry Away

The science and art of obstetric anesthesia has come a long way. Thanks to the techniques of pain relief for labor and delivery available today, mothers-to-be can fully appreciate the wonder of childbirth without the suffering their forebears were obliged to experience.

4

LEAPS AND BOUNDS:
THE WALKING EPIDURAL
AND OTHER ADVANCES

Topics to Be Delivered

- What is a walking epidural, and how does it differ from the standard epidural?
- Medications used for low dose epidurals/spinals
- Which type of technique should you choose?
- The advantages of patient-controlled epidural analgesia

The primary advance made in obstetric anesthesia since I completed my training in 1986 has been the introduction of the walking epidural. The old, classic epidural numbed the lower body completely, immobilizing the woman in the process. By contrast, the walking epidural relieves the pain of labor and delivery while maintaining muscle strength, preserving the ability to walk.

The term "walking epidural" is somewhat of a misnomer. Few women actually walk around after their pain is relieved, not because they are unable to but because most simply prefer to rest in bed. Some women choose to take advantage of their leg strength and walk to the toilet in order to avoid having to use a bedpan. Others utilize their muscle strength to position themselves for delivery, for example, squatting.

Aside from making walking possible, one of the walking epidural's distinct advantages is that it preserves the pelvic and abdominal muscle tone that helps push the baby out during the second stage of labor. The muscle weakness old-fashioned epidurals produced sometimes made this difficult.

The combined effects of pain relief and preserved muscle strength can be achieved with an epidural, a spinal, or a combined spinal-epidural. What matters is not the specific technique but the very low dose of local anesthetic that is used, which maintains muscle function.

Pregnant Pause

Many women fall asleep after getting their epidural, but it's not because medications in the epidural make them sleepy. Rather, it's because their labor pain has prevented them from sleeping—in some cases for a couple of days. Once the pain is eliminated, they are able to get some well-deserved rest so that they can save their energy for the work ahead.

"But will this weak local anesthetic work?" is a common question. The answer is yes, for most women. Even though we now administer only one-half to one-tenth the concentration previously used, we no longer depend on the local anesthetic alone: we mix other types of pain-relieving medications with it. For example, addition of a small dose of narcotic to the low-dose local anesthetic is usually very effective in relieving pain. If pain persists, a higher dose of local anesthetic can easily be added.

THE BENEFIT OF MEDICATION COMBINATION

There is a distinct advantage in administering two or more different types of pain-relieving medication in the epidural or spinal space at the same time. Because the different types of medication act in concert to diminish the pain, the dose of each individual medication can be lowered. Also, because each produces a different type of side effect, and because a relatively small dose of each pain reliever is used, the likelihood of side effects is reduced.

The pain relievers anesthesiologists most commonly combine with local anesthetics are the synthetic narcotics fentanyl and sufentanil, which produce pain relief without muscle weakness. Unlike local anesthetics, narcotics administered into the spinal or epidural space block only the pain nerves, without affecting nerves that control muscle function.

EPIDURAL, SPINAL, OR COMBINED SPINAL-EPIDURAL?

Although spinals and epidurals are used almost interchangeably for childbirth, there are reasons for choosing one over the other. The major factor should be timing—how long it takes for the pain relief to start working, and how long it needs to last. As noted, a spinal begins to relieve labor pain within three to five minutes, as opposed to ten to fifteen minutes with an epidural. But spinal pain relief typically lasts less than two hours, while epidurals can be re-dosed to maintain the pain relief for as long as needed.

Spinals can be made to last a few hours longer by using morphine, a very long-lasting narcotic. In general, though, giving spinal morphine is not as reliable as an epidural for long-lasting pain relief, and it is associated with a higher likelihood of bothersome side effects (itching, nausea, vomiting). Also, spinal morphine does not provide very good pain relief for the second stage of labor. The combined spinal-epidural technique has the best features of both: the spinal component begins to work rapidly, and the epidural catheter can be used to give pain medication for as long as needed.

If you're in relatively early labor and still have hours to go, an epidural makes the most sense because it can last for as long as you may need it. If you don't request pain relief until the end of the first stage of labor or the beginning of the second stage, when delivery is imminent, the difference in onset time between spinals and epidurals becomes a more important factor. In such a situation, it may be advisable to use a spinal, because it will take effect very quickly and you probably won't need the pain relief to last for very long.

A combined spinal-epidural may be an even better choice in this circumstance. Unlike a spinal alone, a combined spinal-epidural enables the administration of additional anesthetics through the epidural catheter, if necessary. So if the labor is prolonged for any reason or if a cesarean is required, as much anesthesia as needed can be added.

Some anesthesiologists advocate use of a combined spinal-epidural early in the first stage of labor. They start by giving a dose through the spinal and then administer the epidural dose as the spinal medication begins to wear off. But if you have hours of labor ahead, I wouldn't advise having a combined spinal-epidural just to get the pain relieved five minutes faster. If your cervix is two to three centimeters dilated, and your obstetrician or midwife has determined that you are truly in labor, I would recommend a low-dose epidural.

The best way to avoid getting yourself into a situation where you need the anesthetic to take effect immediately is to have an epidural catheter inserted early on, before the severe pain begins. The rationale for this approach is made clear in the next chapter.

THE RIGHT AMOUNT

Ideally, you should receive the exact amount of anesthetic necessary to relieve your pain, no more and no less. But it is impossible at the outset to predict the precise amount of medication any particular mother-to-be will require, because everyone has different needs and every labor is unique.

Our approach is to start with a dose that is likely to relieve pain in most, but not necessarily all, women. We then fine-tune pain relief by giving booster doses as needed through the epidural catheter to make you comfortable, or by allowing you to self-administer booster doses. This approach tends to prevent you from receiving more medication than you need. In general, it is easier to add more pain relievers as needed than to wait for an excess to wear off.

PATIENT-CONTROLLED EPIDURAL ANALGESIA (PCEA)

Continuous administration of pain relievers into the epidural space was made possible by electronic pumps that came into use in the 1980s. This technology has had a profound impact on the practice of obstetric anesthesia.

Before these pumps were used, the anesthesiologist would have to keep giving doses of epidural pain medication every so often during labor. By continuously delivering a regulated flow of medication, the pumps solved the problem of the pain that typically occurred between the time one dose wore off and the next began to work. Once started, a pump can deliver medication for the duration of labor and delivery, maintaining constant relief with a low-dose mixture of pain relievers, usually a local anesthetic and a synthetic narcotic, as described above.

Epidural Episodes:
"DON'T GIVE HER TOO MUCH, DOC"

I was called to care for S.G., who was having her first baby. She thought that she wanted an epidural, but was unsure because she had heard a couple of frightening epidural stories. When her labor pain became very intense she decided to ask for an epidural. As I was administering the medication her husband said "Don't give her too much, Doc." His concern that the epidural could be harmful to his wife or their baby, although admirable, was misplaced. Many parents-to-be have expressed these concerns to me. I explain that they shouldn't worry, because with a walking epidural, we administer only a small amount of medication, so it's not dangerous for mother or baby.

Another technological advance was the introduction of programmable pumps that allowed women to control administration of their own pain medication by pushing a button. This can be done in two ways: by allowing the mother-to-be to get booster doses without any "background" flow of medication, or by delivering a low background flow and allowing her to fine-tune the pain control with booster doses. The technique is known as patient-controlled epidural analgesia (PCEA). It has a built-in safety mechanism, as the anesthesiologist sets the maximum amount of medication that the pump will administer. That way, it is not possible for the woman to overdose herself, even if she constantly pushes the button.

Pregnant Pause

Find out if patient-controlled epidural analgesia (PCEA) is available at the hospital where you will be delivering.

PCEA is an excellent way to give epidural medication during labor. Studies have shown that women find this approach more satisfying than when they are not able to dose themselves since they perceive themselves to be—and indeed are—more in control of their situation.

Another advantage of PCEA is that women are more likely to succeed in pushing effectively during the second stage because they tend to retain the feeling of pressure as the baby descends toward the birth canal. By fine-tuning their own medication, they are more likely to give themselves just enough to feel the pressure but not the pain.

Key Concepts to Carry Away

The scientific and technological advances that made walking epidurals (and spinals) possible have revolutionized obstetric anesthesia. Women are now able to be free of the pain of labor and delivery while retaining the muscle strength needed to effectively push the baby out.

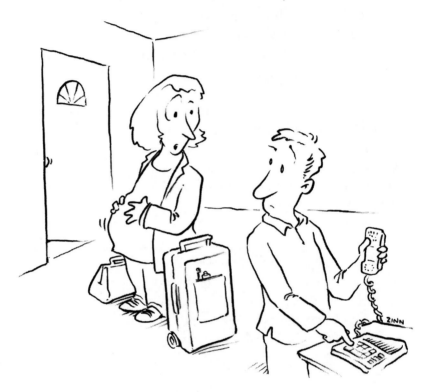

*"When I said call the doctor, I meant the anesthesiologist!
I want my epidural!"*

5

THE TIMING OF LABOR PAIN RELIEF

Topics to Be Delivered

- Is it ever "too early" or "too late" to get an epidural?
- What does the latest research show about "early" epidurals and spinals?
- When should you ask for pain relief?
- Should the pain relief be continued during the second stage of labor?

Many women suffer needlessly for hours in labor because they are led to believe it is either too early or late to get an epidural. The reason? The continuing prevalence of old-fashioned, outdated notions about when epidurals can and should be given. These misconceptions are widely held not only by the women themselves, but even by some obstetric caregivers— doctors, midwives, and nurses alike.

Many people mistakenly believe in the window-of-opportunity concept of pain relief: the idea that there is a specific interval— usually when the cervix is dilated between four and seven centimeters—during which epidurals/spinals can safely be administered. The misguided thinking is that pain relief given "too early" will slow down the progress of labor and may make it necessary to use forceps in the delivery, or even to perform a cesarean. Given too late, the story goes, it may impair the woman's ability to push, or may not take effect rapidly enough to be worthwhile. Neither view has a sound scientific basis.

WHEN IS TOO EARLY?

The "it's too early" idea grew out of research conducted during the 1950s, when the use of regional pain relief was becoming popular. Flawed interpretation of data at that time about the effect of caudal epidurals (see page 22) on the course of labor resulted in the inappropriate recommendation that epidurals be withheld from women in the early stages of labor. This became the practice for generations of obstetrical caregivers, even though epidurals of the 1950s bear little resemblance to those currently used. Again, the concentrations of local anesthetic used for today's walking epidurals are one-fifth to one-tenth the concentrations used fifty years ago.

Pregnant Pause

Can you imagine visiting the dentist to have a tooth drilled, but insisting on not receiving a local anesthetic until *after* the drilling has begun? Sounds absurd, right? Yet this is precisely the approach that most women use for labor pain relief. They wait until the pain becomes unbearable before they get the epidural.

RECENT RESEARCH

On October 1, 1993, the Department of Defense mandated that epidurals be available at military medical hospitals to any laboring woman who wanted one. The results of the new policy, as analyzed at Tripler Army Medical Center in Honolulu, were dramatic. Before epidurals were available on demand, 98 percent of women received systemic (i.v.) narcotics, and only 2 percent received epidurals; when available on demand, 92 percent received epidurals, and only 2 percent received i.v. narcotics.

During one-year intervals before and after epidurals were readily available, researchers tracked what happened to women who got pain relief early—that is, when their cervix was not more than four centimeters dilated. The percentage of forceps deliveries or cesareans was nearly identical during both intervals. In other words, getting an epidural early did not affect the outcome of labor.[5]

A study conducted in Chicago at Northwestern University, and published in 2005, examined the effect of early spinals/epidurals on the progress and outcome of labor in women in spontaneous labor having their first baby. Mothers-to-be who requested pain relief before their cervix was dilated to four centimeters were

Epidural Episodes:
TWENTY-FIRST-CENTURY CARE

P.B. was a twenty-six-year-old first-time mother-to-be who arrived at the labor and delivery suite dilated to two centimeters. When I met her she was walking, or attempting to walk, up and down the hall until contractions made her grab the hand railing, groaning in pain. Her devoted husband massaged her lower back through her hospital gown. I introduced myself and asked whether she had considered an epidural, but got the stock answer: it was "too early" to get relief. I described how the very low doses of anesthetics relieve pain without weakening muscles, meaning she could still walk as much as she wanted. The prospective parents seemed at once confused, suspicious, and hopeful—understandable, given what they had heard before I met them. I spoke with her obstetrician, who agreed with my plan to administer a walking epidural. In twenty minutes she was comfortable. And her husband was as pleased as she at her removal from the agony women have historically endured to the pain-free labor possible today.

given either systemic narcotics or combined spinal-epidural pain relief. Once their cervix reached four centimeters dilation, all women were given patient-controlled epidural analgesia (PCEA; see page 33). The doctors then observed the course of labor and delivery.

The rate of cesarean was nearly identical whether the women received i.v. narcotics or a combined spinal-epidural (21 versus 18 percent, respectively). And labor actually progressed more rapidly if a combined spinal-epidural was given; those women reached full cervical dilation (ten centimeters) an hour and a half sooner than women who received i.v. narcotics. Not surprisingly, the combined spinal-epidural provided better pain relief than did the i.v. narcotics.[6]

The same investigators conducted a follow-up study in 2009 comparing early and late administration of a combined spinal-epidural in first-time mothers-to-be whose labors were being induced. The results were very similar: virtually no difference in the cesarean or forceps rates, and labor a half-hour quicker among women who had the early combined spinal-epidural.[7]

In Israel in 2006, researchers studied the effects of "pure" epidurals (that is, without any spinal component) given either before three or after four centimeters dilation to a group of 449 first-time mothers-to-be. There was no statistically different effect on the rate of forceps (13 percent versus 11 percent) or cesarean delivery (17 percent versus 19 percent); and the time to get to full dilation—ten centimeters—was about thirty minutes less in women given early epidurals.[8]

In a five-year study conducted in China, involving nearly 13,000 first-time mothers-to-be and published in 2009, subjects were randomized to receive an early (one to four centimeters dilation) or late (greater than four centimeters) epidural. Investigators found no difference in the incidence of forceps or cesarean delivery. The time to delivery was not different, regardless of how early the epidural was administered.[9]

Taken together, these studies demonstrate t
or spinals early in labor does not increas
cesarean or forceps delivery, and does n
process of labor; on the contrary, it may speed
confirms what anesthesiologists have been sa
is sensible to give an epidural/spinal early in l

Pregnant Pause

The notion that it's a bad idea to get an epidural early in labor was hatched in the 1950s. It is as false as it is outdated. You should be able to get relief of labor pain at any time. It makes no difference to a woman in labor whether her cervix is two centimeters or six centimeters dilated: pain is pain. You should not be held hostage to your cervix, over whose dilation you have no control.

PAIN AS INDICATOR OF DYSFUNCTIONAL LABOR

Labor is very painful for most women, but if it is dysfunctional, it can hurt even more. Dysfunctional labor means that the cervix dilates at a slower rate than normal, and delivery by forceps or cesarean is more likely. So with dysfunctional labor there is a combination of slow progress and more pain than usual.

The three main causes of dysfunctional labor are inefficient uterine contractions, a large baby, or a small pelvis. Women experiencing it are more likely to request and receive an epidural. But when it turns out that a forceps or cesarean delivery is needed, the epidural is blamed, even though there is no irrefutable evidence that the epidural itself had anything to do with the outcome of labor.

The link between pain and dysfunctional labor was first demonstrated in a 1989 study that showed a correlation between the quality of pain in early labor—before three centimeters' dilation—and the type of delivery that occurred. Sixty-eight percent of women who reported "horrible" or "excruciating" pain during

...ly labor went on to have forceps or cesarean delivery. ...the other hand, only 30 percent of women who rated their pain as "discomforting" went on to have cesarean or forceps delivery. In other words, intense pain very early on in labor was an indicator that labor would be dysfunctional and that forceps or cesarean delivery would be more likely.[10]

Thus, the fact that a woman has pain early on in the process of labor may simply be a sign of dysfunctional labor. Refusing to relieve the pain, even before the cervix is three centimeters dilated, makes no sense.

IS IT EVER TOO LATE?

The misconception that it may be too late to get an epidural has probably been around for as long as epidurals have been used. Since epidurals take awhile to begin working, usually ten to fifteen minutes, they were not considered a good choice for providing pain relief for a woman rapidly approaching the moment of birth.

If anesthesia was needed quickly, for example, for a forceps delivery in a woman who didn't have an epidural catheter in place, what tended to be administered was a type of spinal anesthesia called a "saddle block," which anesthetized the area of that makes contact with a saddle when riding a horse. The advantage of this type of a spinal compared to an epidural was that it worked more quickly, in about three to five minutes. But the relatively high concentration of local anesthetic used for saddle blocks produced profound muscle weakness, making it difficult for the woman to push her baby out.

The introduction of low-dose techniques of spinal anesthesia in the late 1980s changed all this. It became possible to administer a spinal anesthetic that would take effect within three to five minutes and at the same time preserve the muscle strength needed to push effectively. In fact, because of its rapid onset, a low-dose spinal or a combined spinal-epidural is now the procedure of choice when delivery is imminent.

THE OFFICIAL POSITION

The Committee on Obstetric Practice of the American College of Obstetricians and Gynecologists (ACOG) periodically issues committee opinions to advise obstetricians of current thinking on various topics. In June 2006, ACOG published Committee Opinion #339, which addressed head-on the controversial practice of waiting until the cervix was dilated four to five centimeters before giving an epidural:

> ...[I]t has come to the attention of ACOG that some institutions are now requiring that laboring women reach four to five centimeters of cervical dilatation before receiving epidural analgesia...Labor results in severe pain for many women. There is no other circumstance where it is considered acceptable for a person to experience untreated severe pain, amenable to safe intervention, while under a physician's care. In the absence of a medical contraindication, maternal request is a sufficient medical indication for pain relief during labor.[11]

So ACOG comes squarely down on the side of labor pain relief on demand.

WHEN YOU SHOULD ASK FOR PAIN RELIEF

At what point during labor may you ask for pain relief? At what point should you ask? The answers to these questions will be different for every woman and can even vary for the same woman from one labor to the next. If you have decided in advance that you want regional pain relief, I recommend that you have the epidural catheter inserted as soon as your obstetrician or midwife determines you are truly in labor and will be staying in the hospital. I also advise that you have the epidural catheter inserted even if you're not in labor, provided your obstetric caregiver has made a decision to deliver the baby—for example, if your water has broken. You need not wait until the pain begins to have the catheter inserted. Of course, your obstetric caregiver has to be in agreement with this plan.

After the anesthesiologist has inserted the epidural catheter, she or he can hook up the catheter to an electronic infusion pump.

Pregnant Pause

Discuss the issue of the timing of pain relief with your obstetrician or midwife during your pregnancy, so that you can agree on an approach before labor begins.

With the catheter in place, it is a simple matter to turn the pump on, which will then send the pain relieving medication into your epidural space. In this way, you will be all set to receive analgesia when you decide you want it, assuming, of course, that your obstetrician or midwife agrees.

If you wait until you are in severe pain to have the epidural catheter inserted, you've made the situation a bit more difficult for yourself. It is not as easy to remain still while the epidural is being inserted if you are in pain. Keep in mind, also, that the anesthesiologist may not be available at the precise moment you decide that you want pain relief.

Consider how the labor and delivery unit in a hospital functions. Any number of patients may be in various stages of labor just when your pain is becoming unbearable. As minutes start to feel like hours, the anesthesiologist on duty may be busy caring for another woman, and you may have to wait. Remember, too, that an epidural takes ten to fifteen minutes to start working once the medication is injected into the catheter. By far the most sensible option is to have the epidural catheter inserted early, before the severe pain begins.

That said, it is never too late for pain relief. I have administered epidurals and spinals to many women who were dilated to eight, nine or even ten centimeters and were about to begin the second stage of labor, pushing. Patients who receive pain relief in this situation are most appreciative to have been spared the pain of late labor and delivery. Afterward, they often wonder aloud why they had not opted for it earlier.

The important point here is that it is not unreasonable to ask for pain relief even if you are dilated to ten centimeters. If delivery

Epidural Episodes:

BETTER LATE THAN NEVER

J.S. was having her second baby. She had delivered her first baby vaginally, without an epidural, and she was planning to do it the same way this time as well. She bore the pain as her cervix dilated, but when it reached ten centimeters, the trouble began. The baby was not descending properly and because of her intense pain, she was not able to push effectively. Her obstetrician recommended that she assume a squatting position to assist the baby's descent, but her pain prevented her from doing even that. The obstetrician requested that I administer pain relief that would allow effective pushing. I gave J.S. a low-dose spinal. This provided rapid pain relief and preserved her muscle strength so that she could squat and push well. Within an hour she had delivered a beautiful baby. After it was over, her obstetrician remarked that without the spinal, he would have had to perform a cesarean.

is expected to occur within a few minutes it probably is not worthwhile. On the other hand, if the pushing stage lasts for a long time, a spinal/epidural can be enormously beneficial. For women having their first baby, this stage may last two or three hours, or more. There is no way of predicting precisely how long your second stage will last, although your obstetrician or midwife will be able to give you an educated guess. While I am not recommending that you wait until full dilation to ask for it, remember that just because you're far along, doesn't mean that you can't have pain relief.

ALL THE WAY THROUGH

Another important issue about the timing of pain relief is how long to keep it going. Many people are still under the impression that the epidural must be turned off or at least dialed down for the delivery. In some cases, this may be true. If you can't sense any pressure during the second stage as the baby descends, pushing may be more challenging. It is certainly easier to push against something than just to push in the abstract.

Ideally, the epidural (or spinal) will take away the pain sensation but leave you with a sensation of pressure. If you can't feel any pressure sensation at all, then your epidural medication may have to be decreased. As the pain relief begins to wear off, the pressure sensation will return. It's best to begin pushing as you begin to sense the pressure, before the severe pain returns.

Patient-controlled epidural analgesia (PCEA) tends to preserve the pressure sensation, because women in labor give themselves just enough medication to take the pain away without abolishing the pressure sensation that accompanies each contraction. I have found that many mothers-to-be need a boost of a stronger dose of medication as the pushing stage approaches. The controversy regarding turning the pain relief down or even off during the second stage of labor is explored further in chapter 11.

Key Concepts to Carry Away

A woman should receive pain relief when she wants it. She should not have to wait until someone else deems it permissible. Consider a commonsense approach to pain relief. Childbirth hurts, but you can dramatically diminish and perhaps even eliminate the pain by choosing to use a regional pain relief technique. Ideally, you should have the epidural and/or spinal in place before the severe pain starts, so long as labor has been diagnosed, or a decision has been made to deliver the baby. The pain relief should be continued through delivery.

6

EPIDURALS AND SPINALS: A GUIDED TOUR

Topics to Be Delivered

- **Knowing exactly what to expect will reduce anxiety**
- **Why proper positioning is important for a successful epidural/spinal**
- **Step-by-step descriptions of epidural, spinal, and combined spinal-epidural techniques**

What will happen as your anesthesiologist administers your epidural/spinal? Knowing what is coming helps allay any concerns you may have. While the prospect of a needle being inserted into your back is hardly pleasant, perception truly is worse than the reality. Keep in mind that the actual insertion is quick, and that a local anesthetic is used to numb the area beforehand. And remember that the epidural and spinal needles are in place for only a minute or two, just long enough to insert a tiny flexible plastic catheter into the epidural space or to inject medication into the spinal fluid.

MONITORING YOUR VITAL SIGNS

Before you receive your epidural/spinal, as many as three devices will be attached to allow the anesthesiologist to monitor your vital signs. A blood pressure cuff will be placed around your upper arm. Today these cuffs are automatic; a machine has replaced the stethoscope. The first time the device takes your blood pressure, the cuff squeezes your arm very tightly. Don't be surprised by this; subsequent measurements will not feel as tight as the first one. Your heart function may be monitored through small adhesive patches that attach electrocardiogram (EKG) leads to your chest and shoulders. And a pulse oximeter, which resembles a cushioned clothespin, may be placed on one of your fingertips to measure the amount of oxygen in your blood. Your baby's heart rate may also be monitored while the epidural/spinal is being inserted.

POSITIONING IS IMPORTANT

Next, to make your epidural/spinal space as accessible as possible for the anesthesiologist, you will be positioned in one of two ways, either sitting or lying on your side (figure 6-1). The purpose of both positions is the same: to help you round out

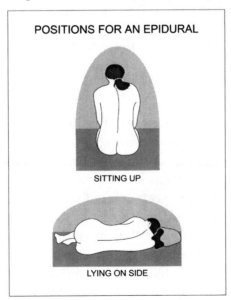

Fig. 6-1. *The two positions used for insertion of epidurals and spinals.*

48

your lower back as much as possible. The outwardly curved position of your lower back increases the opening between the spinous processes, the little bumps you can feel running down the center of your back. This widening makes it much easier for your anesthesiologist to direct the epidural/spinal needle to the desired location (figure 6-2).

If you are in a sitting position, you will be asked to dangle your arms in front of you, which relaxes your shoulders forward and helps you push your lower back out. If you are lying on your side, you will be asked to curl into a fetal position. Do your best, but in either position, we understand it is challenging to curl up and bring your knees to your chest with a pregnant abdomen in the way!

One more point about the position you'll be asked to get into: Don't try to tuck your neck down into your chest. Doing so doesn't help at all to round out your lower back, and it can cause a nasty neck ache afterward.

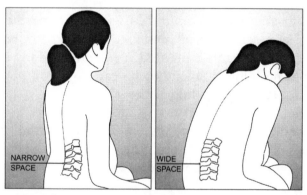

Fig. 6-2. *The effect of a rounded lower back on the spaces between the spinous processes. Note how the distance between the spinous processes widens when the back is rounded out. This is important, since the epidural/spinal needle must pass between the spinal processes.*

CLEANING AND NUMBING

Once you are in position, your back will be cleansed with an antiseptic solution. Because this solution is at room temperature, it feels cold when applied to your skin. After your skin has been cleansed, the anesthesiologist will place a drape over your back. The drape has a hole in it, to allow access to the area where the epidural/spinal needle will be inserted.

Just before the anesthesiologist inserts the epidural/spinal needle, he or she will numb a small area of skin by injecting a local anesthetic. Most women later tell me the skin numbing was the only painful part of the entire epidural or spinal procedure. To keep things in perspective, remember this: after having their epidural/spinal placed, most women say it hurt less than having their i.v. inserted.

Pregnant Pause

When administering an epidural/spinal, I tell mothers-to-be the procedure is about as painful as having an i.v. inserted. Most women say afterward that the i.v. hurt more.

FINALLY—YOU'RE READY

After your skin has been numbed with local anesthetic, you should feel a sensation of pressure, but not pain, when the epidural/spinal needle is inserted. If you do sense any pain, tell your anesthesiologist so she or he can give you more local anesthetic before proceeding further.

The anesthesiologist depends on feedback from you for guidance. By the same token, your anesthesiologist should explain every step of the procedure so you are not surprised by anything that occurs.

Next comes the most demanding part of the procedure for your anesthesiologist; the actual insertion of the tip of the needle into the epidural or spinal space. The technique is based on feel, since it is not possible to see the epidural or spinal space, and on skill attained through experience.

For an epidural, once the needle tip is in position, a tiny catheter is threaded through it into the epidural space. The catheter is a

50

thin, flexible tube with one to three holes at its tip through which anesthetic medication is injected. If it brushes against a nerve root as it passes in, you may experience a "funny-bone" sensation in your back, hip, or leg. Although this is uncomfortable, it passes quickly, and is no cause for alarm. With the newer, more flexible epidural catheters, the likelihood of experiencing this sensation has been reduced.

Pregnant Pause

As soon as the epidural catheter is inserted, the needle is removed. For the rest of labor, the only thing in your back will be three or four inches of the epidural catheter. You can lie on it and move around freely without worry.

After the epidural catheter is inserted, your anesthesiologist will remove the needle, leaving three or four of inches of catheter within your epidural space. Then he or she will secure the catheter to your back with adhesive tape. Having an epidural catheter in place will not prevent you from lying on your back or moving around. You do not have to worry about its becoming dislodged unintentionally. Although this can occur, it is unlikely and easily remedied. For a spinal, once the needle is inserted, anesthetic medication will be injected into the spinal fluid, and then the needle will be removed.

Pregnant Pause

It's not possible to know from sensation alone whether you are being given a spinal, an epidural, or a combined spinal-epidural. Once your skin is numbed, you should only feel pressure in your lower back during any of the procedures.

If you are given a combined spinal-epidural, the epidural needle is placed in the epidural space, and then a spinal needle is passed through the epidural needle and the dura to reach the spinal fluid. After the anesthetic medication is injected, the spinal needle is withdrawn and a catheter is threaded through the epidural needle into the epidural space. The epidural needle is then withdrawn and the catheter is secured to your back with adhesive tape, as described above. Having worked with thousands of patients, and having undergone spinal anesthesia myself, I can assure you that the procedure really isn't very painful.

Key Concepts to Carry Away

Keep an open mind about your pain relief options. The thought of getting an epidural/spinal tends to be much worse than the procedure itself, which for most women causes less discomfort than a single uterine contraction.

7

IF YOUR DELIVERY IS CESAREAN

Topics to Be Delivered

- **The difference between planned, urgent, and emergency cesareans**
- **Anesthetic choices for cesarean**
- **Why regional anesthesia is preferred for cesarean**
- **The risks of general anesthesia**
- **What will occur in the operating room?**
- **The importance of focusing on the big picture**

Nearly one of every three babies in the United States is born by cesarean delivery. Some cesareans are planned long before labor actually begins. Unplanned cesareans, decided on once labor is under way, have different degrees of urgency. For example, if a baby is discovered to be in the breech position rather than head-first, a cesarean may be called for, but the situation is not necessarily an emergency. But if the fetal heart rate slows and does not recover, an extremely urgent or "stat" (from statim, Latin for "immediately") cesarean is required. The type of anesthesia chosen is largely determined by the urgency of the situation.

GENERAL VERSUS REGIONAL ANESTHESIA

Today, more than 90 percent of planned cesareans in the United States are performed using regional anesthesia (epidurals/ spinals). Until the 1970s–1980s, general anesthesia was the technique of choice for cesarean delivery in hospitals nation-wide. Its use began to decline as its drawbacks for baby and mother became increasingly clear:

- The general anesthetics that produce unconsciousness in the mother pass through the placenta and may also cause the baby to be born sleepy and breathing too slowly. If this occurs, the newborn may require assistance breathing until the effects of the general anesthetics wear off.

- For general anesthesia, a breathing tube must be inserted into the windpipe (trachea). During this procedure, known as intubation, it is possible for residual food or liquid in the stomach to be vomited and spilled into the lungs (aspirated). Aspiration does not happen with regional anes-thesia because when we're awake, our gag reflex prevents it.

- With general anesthesia the mother is not awake to enjoy the birth of her baby.

On the other hand, it is important to bear in mind that except in rare cases, general anesthesia is a safe, reliable method for women who want or need it. The anesthesiologist will maximize the chance of a successful intubation, and the pediatrician can help the newborn breathe if necessary. In some situations, general anesthesia may be the only option. Regional anesthesia cannot be used if:

- The baby has a dangerously slow heart rate and a stat cesarean delivery becomes necessary, with no time to spare. In most cases, it takes less time to give general anesthesia than to give an epidural/spinal. But in some circumstances, for example, if an epidural catheter is already in place and being used to provide labor pain relief, it is a simple matter for the anesthesiologist to inject additional medication through the catheter, allowing the obstetrician to proceed with the cesarean.

Epidural Episodes:

IN A FLASH

A.F. was in labor with her first baby. She was not sure that she wanted an epidural, and was using breathing techniques to deal with the pain of her contractions. Her cervix was dilated five centimeters when her nurse noticed that the baby's heart rate was slowing. It had been 130 to 140 beats per minute, but it was now 70 to 80 beats per minute, and wasn't improving. Her obstetrician was notified immediately, and he decided to quickly bring A.F. to the cesarean section room. I was paged stat and while her bed was being rolled down the hall, I assured A.F. that we would do our very best to see that she and her baby would be fine. I gave her general anesthesia and three minutes later her obstetrician delivered the baby. Fortunately, mother and baby did very well and they both went home four days later. General anesthesia was key in this case, as it made possible rapid delivery of the baby.

- The mother-to-be has substantial bleeding that causes her blood pressure to fall. Since the doses of anesthetics used for cesareans done under epidurals/spinals have a tendency to lower blood pressure, general anesthesia is probably a better choice in this circumstance.

- There is a skin infection on the lower back. The needle could transport bacteria from the skin into the epidural or spinal space, causing a serious infection such as an epidural abscess or meningitis.

- There is a bleeding disorder. If the blood does not clot normally, and the epidural/spinal needle nicks a vein, excessive bleeding may occur in the epidural or spinal space. This could cause permanent damage to nerves in the area if the problem is not recognized and quickly corrected.

- If the mother-to-be refuses to have a needle inserted into her back.

Pregnant Pause

In some circumstances, general anesthesia is necessary for cesarean. Although regional anesthesia is usually preferred, general anesthesia has a long and increasingly excellent safety record, and should be no cause for concern.

REGIONAL PAIN RELIEF: CESAREAN VERSUS LABOR

The dose of local anesthetic required for spinals/epidurals for cesareans is much higher than that for relieving labor pain. This higher anesthetic concentration will make you quite numb, and because it affects muscle function, you should expect your legs to feel weak. In fact, you may not be able to move them for a few hours after the operation. Odd as it may feel, this loss of muscle function is expected, temporary, and not dangerous.

But again, if an unanticipated situation during labor requires an emergency cesarean and an epidural catheter is already in place, general anesthesia can usually be avoided with a booster of stronger local anesthetic. In this way, you are awake for the arrival of your baby, who like you will have avoided the risks of general anesthesia noted above.

It's especially important to have an epidural catheter in place in situations known to be associated with a greater chance of forceps, vacuum, or cesarean delivery. For women who are planning vaginal delivery of twins or who are attempting to deliver vaginally after a previous cesarean, I strongly recommend the placement of an epidural catheter early in the course of labor.

WHICH REGIONAL WILL IT BE?

If you receive regional anesthesia for your cesarean, will it be spinal, epidural, or combined spinal-epidural? If you happen to have an epidural catheter already in place for labor, your anesthesiologist will likely continue with the epidural by simply injecting a higher dose of local anesthetic through the catheter. If your cesarean is planned, most anesthesiologists in the United States prefer to use a spinal. Some may favor an epidural, and others will use a combined spinal-epidural technique.

As discussed in chapter 4, each technique has its advantages and disadvantages, and there is no one right way. A spinal takes effect more rapidly than an epidural. While this may not make a difference for a planned cesarean, if you need an urgent or emergency cesarean, saving a few minutes may be important. But a spinal lasts only as long as a single dose of anesthetic. Epidurals can be made to last indefinitely, because extra doses of medication can be injected through the catheter as needed. And again, the epidural catheter can be left in place to provide pain relief after the cesarean. A combined spinal-epidural technique has both advantages: the anesthesia takes effect rapidly, and there is an option to give additional doses of anesthetics, if necessary.

A STEP-BY-STEP TOUR OF THE CESAREAN EXPERIENCE

When you are brought into the operating room, you will probably immediately notice that the room is very cold. It is common hospital practice to keep operating rooms cold so that the surgeons, who wear surgical gowns over their scrub suits, will be comfortable. The problem is that you, the patient, are wearing only a thin hospital gown with an embarrassingly open back. Short of insisting the entire operating room be warmed, which may not be such a bad idea, you can ask to be covered with warm blankets—except for your abdomen, of course, where the incision will be made.

After you are positioned on the operating table, the monitoring devices discussed in chapter 6 will be put into place: a blood pressure cuff around your arm, EKG leads on your chest and shoulders, and a pulse oximeter on your finger. Your anesthesiologist will use these devices throughout the cesarean to monitor your vital signs (i.e., blood pressure, pulse, heart rhythm, and the amount of oxygen in your blood).

GOING GENERAL

If you are to receive general anesthesia, an oxygen mask will be placed over your nose and mouth. You will be instructed to take some deep breaths to fill your lungs completely with pure oxygen before going to sleep. Anesthetics will then be administered through your i.v. line to rapidly make you sleepy. Once you are asleep, the anesthesiologist will place a breathing tube in your trachea, or windpipe, to provide oxygen and anesthetic gases during the operation. As soon as the cesarean is completed, the anesthesiologist will awaken you and immediately remove the breathing tube. Very few people have any recollection of the breathing tube at all; the only indication it was there may be a mildly sore throat for a day or so.

THE REGIONAL ROUTE

If regional anesthesia is used, you will be positioned for the insertion of an epidural/spinal in your lower back, unless an epidural catheter was already placed for labor. A drop in blood pressure, which is unlikely with the low dosage of medication used for labor, is more common with the higher dose used for cesareans. Your anesthesiologist is well aware of this, and will be ready to promptly treat any fall in blood pressure with intravenous fluids and medications. Do not be surprised if you experience a temporary feeling of lightheadedness or nausea as your body adapts to the anesthetic.

Before the cesarean actually begins, the obstetrician will hang a surgical drape between your chest and abdomen. This drape will prevent you from watching the operation being performed. You may be given oxygen to breathe through either a clear mask or plastic prongs positioned in your nostrils.

Before your surgery starts, your anesthesiologist will test the skin of your abdomen to ensure that the anesthesia is working properly and that you are numb. Do not be surprised if you feel a sensation of pressure during this test; this is normal. Local anesthetics block the sensation of pain, but not sensations of pressure.

The sensation you will feel during the cesarean is similar to what you feel while having a tooth drilled at the dentist's office. After your tooth is numbed with local anesthetic, you do not feel pain from the drilling, but you can still feel some pressure on your teeth and gums as the dentist works. Likewise, during the cesarean, you will feel pressure in different parts of your abdomen and chest. If the sensation bothers you, or if you feel any pain, tell your anesthesiologist so she or he can administer additional medication to make you comfortable.

Pregnant Pause

Many women are frightened that the anesthesia won't work and that they will feel the surgery. Don't worry. Before the cesarean starts your abdomen will be tested to be sure that it is completely numb.

Your arms will be placed out of the way, so that they do not interfere with the surgery. Most commonly, they are positioned on two armrests attached to either side of the operating table. It is important that you resist any temptation to touch your abdomen during the surgery, as this would contaminate the sterile area. Some anesthesiologists loosely wrap adhesive tape around patients' arms as a reminder to keep them on the armrests. Before your cesarean is started, your obstetrician will check your abdomen once again to make sure you are completely numb. Your obstetrician will begin the cesarean only after confirming that the anesthesia is working well.

THE BIRTH

In most hospitals, when regional anesthesia is used, the spouse or partner is seated at the head of the operating table to provide support and to share in the experience of the birth. By contrast, during general anesthesia, it is the policy of most hospitals that only the surgical team be present in the room, since the support person's assistance is of no benefit with the mother unconscious. Also, the presence of a non-medical person may make it more difficult for everyone to focus on his or her job: caring for the anesthetized mother and for the newborn.

Your baby will be born a few minutes after the beginning of the cesarean operation. If you have regional anesthesia, your obstetrician may give you a glimpse of your baby as soon as she or he is born. Your baby will then be cleaned up, examined, wrapped in a blanket, and laid in your arms. If you have general anesthesia, you will first meet your baby when you are awakened, as soon as the cesarean is completed.

AFTER THE BIRTH

After your baby is born, the obstetrician will close your incision in layers, working from the uterus to the skin. During this interval, some women are greatly aided by a mild sedative such as midazolam (Versed), which makes it easier to remain relaxed while the operation is completed.

REALITY CHECK: IF YOU NEED A CESAREAN

Nearly one-third of all babies in the United States are delivered by cesarean, and that number is steadily rising. So it should not surprise you if you end up with a cesarean despite plans to the contrary. In some countries the rates are much higher. In China, for example, the cesarean rate is nearly 50 percent, and in private hospitals in some sections of Brazil, the rate exceeds 80 percent.

Over the years, I have noticed that many women planning to deliver vaginally feel as though they have somehow failed if they need a cesarean. Their perception of failure is a result of bias that leads women to believe that vaginal delivery is good and cesarean is bad. Attitudes among women and obstetricians on this subject are changing, and cesareans by choice are gaining acceptance. In any case, it's important to keep in mind that a cesarean is just another—not a "worse"—way to have a baby.

Key Concepts to Carry Away

Modern anesthesia has helped to make cesarean delivery a comfortable, exciting, and fulfilling experience. Understanding your anesthetic options for cesarean will make the entire process less intimidating.

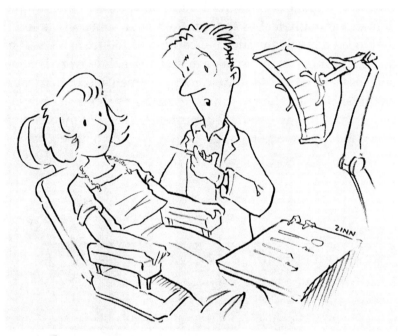

"Let me see if I have this right—you don't want me to give you the local anesthesia until **after** I've started the drilling?"

8

IT AIN'T OVER TILL IT'S OVER: POSTPARTUM PAIN RELIEF

Topics to Be Delivered

- **Contractions after delivery**
- **Pain after vaginal delivery**
- **Pain after cesarean delivery**
- **Systemic pain relievers for postpartum pain**
- **Epidural/spinal techniques for postpartum pain**

Unfortunately, the pain of childbirth does not end the moment your baby is born. Postpartum contractions of the uterus, known as after-pains, occur following both vaginal and cesarean delivery. And other pain is more specific to the type of delivery you have. Following vaginal delivery, the pain is centered in the vaginal and/or perineal area. After cesarean delivery, pain is sensed mainly in the surgical wound.

AFTER-PAINS

Immediately after the baby and placenta are delivered, the uterus contracts vigorously as it begins shrinking back to its pre-pregnancy size. These contractions are essential because as the uterus gets smaller, it helps stop bleeding from the area where the placenta was attached. But the cramping pains can be severe, and tend to get worse with each successive delivery. For women who have had many babies, postpartum contractions can hurt more than labor.

Pregnant Pause

Although often not taken very seriously by health care providers, after-pains can be quite severe. For some mothers, the after-pains are even worse than the pain of labor itself.

To make matters worse, Pitocin, a medication routinely given as soon as the placenta is delivered to help the uterus contract, intensifies after-pains; and administration of the drug continues for a few hours after delivery to minimize blood loss. During breast-feeding, oxytocin, the body's natural form of Pitocin, is released from the mother's pituitary gland, causing the after-pains to become very strong. One patient who had three previous deliveries told me she did not intend to breast-feed her fourth child because she remembered the awful after-pains nursing had caused with her last baby. I explained that fear of after-pains should not be the reason to avoid breast-feeding, since the pain can be treated using oral medications or, even better, by continuing an epidural after delivery. Although it is not usually considered, much less done, you may want to ask your anesthesiologist and obstetrician about this option.

PAIN AFTER VAGINAL DELIVERY

The pain after vaginal delivery varies considerably. Women who have had an easy delivery may experience only mild soreness, while the pain can be quite severe among those for whom delivery was difficult. Postpartum pain tends to be worse if forceps or vacuum were used, if an episiotomy was done, or if the tissues of the vagina, perineum, and anus and/or rectum were torn.

Evidence now shows that an episiotomy, a controlled surgical incision of the perineum once routinely done to limit tissue injury during delivery, is usually unnecessary. As a result, few obstetricians perform episiotomies nowadays, except in specific situations, for example, just before a forceps delivery. Regardless, if the tissues of your perineum are injured, you will have postpartum pain. You may also experience other types of pain after vaginal delivery. Hemorrhoids, for example, a common occurrence during pregnancy, are often aggravated by childbirth.

PAIN AFTER CESAREAN

If you have a cesarean, the postoperative pain can be severe. In addition to the comparatively dull ache of uterine contractions, you may feel a sharp or burning pain from the incision itself. Some women also notice that their shoulders hurt, a condition caused by irritation of the lining of the upper abdomen by blood, amniotic fluid, and/or air within the abdominal cavity. This shoulder pain usually disappears within the first twenty-four hours after delivery.

THE IMPORTANCE OF POSTPARTUM PAIN RELIEF

As is true of labor pain, postpartum pain can be harmful to mother and newborn. If you are in pain, you will not be able to interact with your newborn as well as you would like.

Unrelieved pain can also lead to medical complications. For example, if pain after a cesarean prevents you from moving around and getting out of bed, you are more likely to develop pneumonia from not breathing deeply, and to develop blood clots from poor circulation. So, in addition to avoiding unnecessary suffering, there are good medical reasons for you to relieve your postpartum pain. And you can—without harming your child.

AFTER-PAIN MEDICATION AND YOUR NEWBORN

If you are nursing, any systemic (i.v. or oral) medication you take gets passed on through your breast milk. Although this is a relatively tiny percentage of the dose you receive, a newborn can be affected because he or she is so small. If you become drowsy from taking narcotic pain relievers, your breast-feeding baby is likely to be sleepy as well.

Epidurals/spinals, meanwhile, make as much sense for postpartum pain as they do for labor pain. Because a smaller dose of medication is given with regional techniques, less is passed to the newborn through your breast milk. If your delivery did not cause significant tearing of your vaginal or perineal tissues, the pain may be relatively mild and you may get by with small doses of systemic pain relievers like Tylenol or Motrin.

SYSTEMIC NARCOTICS AND PCA

The standard method of treating postoperative pain has historically been to inject narcotics like morphine or Demerol into a thigh or arm muscle every few hours. But the delay between the request for pain medication and the time it begins to take effect makes the technique inefficient, and less than ideal.

Intravenous patient-controlled analgesia (PCA), popularized in the late 1980s, avoids that delay by allowing you to push a button connected to an electronic pump that triggers a narcotic injection directly into your vein, eliminating both the time once required to call and have the nurse bring the medication and the time needed for the medication to travel from muscle to brain. Because the narcotic is injected directly into your bloodstream, it reaches your brain very rapidly. The pump, the same type used for patient-controlled epidural analgesia, is programmed so that you cannot overdose yourself. For example, if the pump is set for a maximum of one dose every ten minutes, it will not give you more than that, even if you push the button every minute. And if the narcotic makes you too drowsy to push the button, you will not be able to give yourself any more doses—another built-in safety mechanism.

Pregnant Pause

Patient-controlled analgesia (PCA) frees the patient from dependence on nurses, who are frequently busy caring for other patients at the same time. An additional benefit is that the freedom to manage one's own pain is empowering.

In many hospitals, pain after cesarean is routinely treated with i.v. PCA narcotics. Although the method is clearly better than the old-fashioned way of having a nurse inject the narcotics into a muscle, the disadvantages of systemic narcotics still apply: relatively poor pain relief and a high likelihood of side effects.

EPIDURAL/SPINAL NARCOTICS AFTER CESAREAN

Some hospitals use a regional approach to provide pain relief after a cesarean. In these hospitals, the most common practice is to give a narcotic such as morphine (Duramorph) into the epidural or spinal space. Among the drugs used, morphine is the longest-lasting. A small dose of epidural/spinal morphine given at the time of a cesarean can provide pain relief for as long as twenty-four hours.

Pregnant Pause

The most common side effect of epidural/spinal morphine is itching. If you experience it, your anesthesiologist can treat it with a medication such as Narcan. Giving small doses of Narcan will reverse the narcotic side effects and only minimally, if at all, affect the pain relief the narcotics provide.

Drawbacks to epidural/spinal morphine may include itching, nausea, vomiting, drowsiness, and, potentially, slow breathing. Other narcotics such as fentanyl and sufentanil are less likely to have these effects. But the pain relief does not last very long—only two to three hours—so these narcotics are best given repeatedly though an epidural catheter, using PCEA.

PATIENT-CONTROLLED EPIDURAL ANALGESIA AFTER CESAREAN

PCEA is an excellent technique of providing pain relief after cesarean. The epidural catheter is left in place after the operation, delivering a continuous infusion of pain relievers and enabling the mother to self-administer a "booster dose" by pushing a button. The most severe pain occurs in the first day or two following the procedure, so it's a good idea to use PCEA for approximately forty-eight hours.

An ideal pain-relieving mixture to use for PCEA after cesarean contains a small dose of a local anesthetic combined with a small dose of narcotic. This combination provides excellent pain relief without compromising muscle strength, which is the same principle used for the walking epidural. Unlike women who have the walking epidural during labor but usually prefer to rest in bed, women who have had a cesarean are encouraged to get up and walk around. The epidural pump can travel with you (figure 3-5), since it is mounted on wheels and attached to the pole on which the i.v. fluid bag is hung. PCEA combines the advantages of excellent pain relief, minimal side effects, and awake and alert mothers who can control their own dosing.

PCEA AFTER VAGINAL DELIVERY

Severe after-pains from uterine contractions and/or significant injury to perineal tissues may cause pain that cannot adequately be treated with oral pain relievers. In these situations I recommend leaving the epidural catheter in place for a day or two to provide pain relief with PCEA. The contraction pains during labor are best relieved by epidurals, so why not relieve postpartum contraction pains the same way?

Take the case of a woman delivering her third or fourth baby, who, following her last delivery, experienced after-pains more

K.V. was a first-time mother who elected to have epidural pain relief. She delivered a baby boy as large as he was beautiful—weighing in at 8 lbs 14 oz. K.V. was 5'2" and had a petite build. So it was not surprising that she ended up with a tear in her perineum, expertly repaired by her obstetrician immediately after the delivery. Knowing that such an injury hurts considerably, I proposed that K.V. leave the epidural catheter in place and use PCEA for pain control. She was very pleased with the epidural she had during labor, and readily agreed to the suggestion. So for the next two days, she received PCEA, which prevented pain without making her sleepy. Three hours before she was scheduled to go home we removed the epidural catheter, stopping the flow of medication. By the time she was discharged she certainly felt the difference—but thanks to the PCEA, she never experienced the level of pain she would have in those first forty-eight hours.

severe than her labor. If we relieve her pain of labor and delivery with an epidural, why would we then remove the epidural as soon as she delivers? Although it makes no sense, that is routine practice nationwide. Similarly, injury to the tissue of the vagina and perineum can be very painful, so leaving the epidural in place and using it to provide PCEA is a very sensible approach.

Pregnant Pause

Although PCEA is an excellent means for treating pain after cesarean, it is not routinely used at most hospitals. You should find out what type of pain relief is available at your hospital before you deliver, by asking your obstetrical caregiver and an anesthesiologist.

Every technique has its drawbacks. After delivery, some women are bothered by having the catheter in their back and being hooked up to an epidural pump. And at some institutions, hospital policy may not allow them to shower if an epidural catheter is in place. Still, most women I care for are so pleased with the quality of pain relief they receive from PCEA, they willingly put up with the inconvenience.

Key Concepts to Carry Away

Although it's not much discussed, there may also be considerable pain after delivery. Like the pain of childbirth, it can and should be treated. Safe and effective regional pain relief techniques may be used to make you comfortable even after you've had your baby.

9

THE RISKS OF EPIDURALS AND SPINALS

Topics to Be Delivered

- Headaches after epidurals/spinals
- Low blood pressure caused by epidurals/spinals
- Effects of epidurals/spinals on your baby's heart rate
- Rare side effects of epidurals/spinals

For the overwhelming majority of patients, epidurals/spinals are safe for both mother and baby. But there are risks associated with all medical procedures, and epidurals/spinals are no exception. No procedure is 100 percent guaranteed. Problems can and do occur occasionally, resulting in complications that can have short-term or, rarely, long-lasting after-effects. You need to understand the risks and benefits involved so that you can make an informed decision about using an epidural or spinal.

Keep in mind that among potential side effects, those that are most typical are easily dealt with and not long-lasting. Serious side effects are rare. Far more common yet virtually never discussed are the risks of *not* choosing an epidural/spinal for childbirth, as you'll learn in the next chapter.

Before performing the epidural/spinal, your anesthesiologist will discuss the procedure with you. He or she will then have you sign a consent form that details the risks involved. The problem is that it's difficult to concentrate on these important issues when you are in the throes of excruciating labor pain. It is much better to carefully consider the risks and benefits of epidurals/spinals long before your labor begins.

Pregnant Pause

Epidurals and spinals offer many benefits and are relatively safe procedures, but it's possible that complications may occur. You should have a thorough understanding of their benefits as well as their risks so that you can make an informed choice about what is right for you.

RISK: SORENESS AT THE SITE OF INSERTION

One of the most common complaints about epidurals/spinals after delivery is soreness or tenderness in the lower back at the place where the needle was inserted. The discomfort, like a bruise from hitting your shin on a piece of furniture, usually fades away in a couple of days and may be treated with a mild analgesic like Tylenol or Motrin. Some patients find that a heating pad is also helpful.

Most women do not even notice this discomfort. They simply may not have it, or other aches and pains may be bothering them more, such as soreness of the perineum or breast engorgement.

RISK: SPINAL HEADACHE

Headaches caused by epidurals/spinals are collectively known as spinal headaches or post-dural puncture headaches. The terms are synonymous. Although headache is the most common complication of epidurals and spinals, keep in mind that the chance of getting one is approximately 1 to 2 percent. While a spinal headache can be quite painful, the good news is it can be treated. To understand the treatment, you first have to understand what causes the headache.

Spinal headaches are caused by leakage of spinal fluid, a clear liquid surrounding the brain and spinal cord that is kept in place by a layer of tissue called the dura (figure 3-1). When an epidural/spinal needle creates a hole in the dura, the fluid may leak out into the epidural space, and a headache may result.

Pregnant Pause

The chance of getting a headache as a result of an epidural/spinal is small—about 1 or 2 percent. Although they can be very painful, spinal headaches can also be effectively and quickly treated. Just inform your anesthesiologist so that she or he can take care of it.

Why is the chance of getting a headache so low? The likelihood is directly related to the size of the hole in the dura. With an epidural, there is usually no hole at all, as your anesthesiologist makes every attempt to avoid puncturing the dura with the needle. Despite best efforts, however, it still happens to between one and two of 100 women who undergo the procedure. Since the diameter of the epidural needle must be large enough to allow passage of the epidural catheter, the hole it can create in the dura is also relatively large, and usually results in a headache.

For spinal techniques, your anesthesiologist will intentionally pass the needle through the dura, so there is no avoiding creating a hole. But the spinal needle has a very small diameter because it only has to accommodate an injection of liquid medication, not a catheter. So the hole made in the dura is relatively small, and not likely to produce a headache—again, only about 1 to 2 percent of the time.

Another reason for the low headache incidence has to do with the pencil-point shape of the spinal needle tips that have been in use since the mid-1980s. Fluid is much less likely to leak through the hole produced by a needle of this shape. The actual diameters of epidural and spinal needles are shown in figure 9-1.

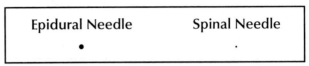

| Epidural Needle | Spinal Needle |

Fig. 9-1. *Actual size of the diameters of epidural and spinal needles shown in cross-section.*

Spinal headaches range from mild to severe. The pain may be located in the front, back, or side of the head. A mild headache may be bothersome, but a severe headache may prevent you from going about your normal routine.

A unique feature of spinal headaches is that they are related to your position. The pain is always worsened when you sit or stand, and tends to intensify the longer you hold your head upright; lying down relieves the headache almost immediately. If the pain does not change with your position, the headache is likely due to some cause other than the epidural/spinal.

Pregnant Pause

Post-dural puncture (spinal) headaches are made worse by sitting upright or standing; they are relieved by lying down. If your headache does not go away when you lie down, it is highly unlikely that the epidural or spinal was the cause.

Left untreated, spinal headaches usually disappear on their own within one to two weeks, as the hole in the dura heals. If the headache is mild it will likely resolve in a few days, so if the mother has assistance at home, enabling her to spend a good amount of time resting in bed, I usually recommend a wait-and-see approach. But for the many women who will be busy caring for their newborn and, possibly, older children as well, treatment is necessary. If a woman cannot remain in bed, or if the headache is severe, I may recommend an epidural blood patch.

TREATMENT OF SPINAL HEADACHE:
EPIDURAL BLOOD PATCH

To perform an epidural blood patch, the anesthesiologist draws approximately half an ounce of blood from a vein in the arm and injects it into the epidural space. The blood forms a clot, which acts as a patch to plug the hole in the dura. The blood patch prevents spinal fluid from leaking out, and this relieves the symptoms of the headache (figure 9-2). Eventually, the blood clot dissolves, but by that time, your dura will have healed, closing the hole. For nearly all patients, the headache goes away as soon as the blood is injected.

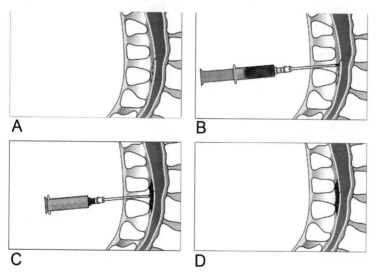

Fig. 9-2. *Epidural blood patch.* **A**: *Spinal fluid leaking through hole in dura.* **B**: *Epidural needle tip positioned in epidural space with patient's own blood in attached syringe.* **C**: *Blood being injected into epidural space.* **D**: *Blood forming clot over hole in dura, preventing further leakage of spinal fluid.*

Although the epidural blood patch works immediately in nearly everyone, for approximately one in four patients the headache returns in a day or two, This is probably caused by the blood clot "slipping" out of position so that it no longer is plugging the hole in the dura. If this happens, a second blood patch may be done. Some patients choose this option, but others may not want it since, by then, they are one day closer to the dura having healed itself.

Pregnant Pause

An epidural blood patch can cure a severe spinal headache. If the headache is relatively mild and the new mother is able to rest at home, a blood patch may not be necessary, since even a severe headache usually gets better on its own within one to two weeks. If you happen to get a spinal headache, you should discuss your circumstances and treatment options with your anesthesiologist.

RISK: LOW BLOOD PRESSURE

Local anesthetics injected into the epidural or spinal space may lower the mother's blood pressure. A slight decrease in pressure is not a problem. In fact, blood pressure after an epidural/spinal is generally closer to what it was before labor started, because when you're in pain, your blood pressure rises. Take the pain away, and your blood pressure returns to its normal level.

But blood pressure that is too low can cause problems. You may feel light-headed or nauseated. More important, the lowered blood pressure may reduce the blood flow to the placenta, which in turn reduces the amount of oxygen delivered to the baby.

The high-dose epidurals formerly used during labor and delivery were known for causing the mother's blood pressure to fall. To counter this anticipated effect, anesthesiologists routinely gave the mother fluids through her i.v. before administering the epidural. If the blood pressure fell despite this precaution, more intravenous fluids and medications were administered to increase blood pressure. This is still done for the higher-dose epidurals and spinals used to provide anesthesia for cesareans.

Unlike high-dose epidurals and spinals, currently used low-dose walking epidurals/spinals do not usually produce a significant fall in the mother's blood pressure. This is because the low-dose methods take effect relatively slowly, over ten to fifteen minutes, giving the body time to adapt and minimizing any effect on blood pressure. As a result, many anesthesiologists no longer administer i.v. fluid before the epidural, saving time and trouble.

I recall many patients in the "old days" who were in severe pain but whose epidurals were delayed because they had not yet received enough intravenous fluid. Also, a lot of fluid given through the i.v. ends up in the bladder, producing the need to urinate frequently.

Pregnant Pause

Low blood pressure can reduce blood flow, and therefore oxygen supply, to the baby. The low-dose epidurals/spinals used for labor today are unlikely to decrease blood pressure; but just in case, your blood pressure will be checked frequently and your baby's heart rate will be monitored continuously. If a fall in your blood pressure does occur, it can be corrected rapidly.

POSITION IS EVERYTHING

Whether or not an epidural/spinal is in place, pregnant women may experience low blood pressure when they lie flat on their backs. The fall in blood pressure may cause them to feel light-headed, flushed, and shaky. This circumstance, known as supine hypotensive syndrome, may occur once the baby becomes heavy enough to compress two of the mother's major blood vessels, the aorta and the vena cava. When they are compressed, blood flow is temporarily blocked, which causes the blood pressure to fall. That is why beginning in mid-pregnancy right through labor you are advised not to lie flat on your back, but rather on your side.

RISK: SPINALS/EPIDURALS AND BRADYCARDIA

It is normal for the baby's heart rate to speed up and slow down during the course of labor, whether or not the mother has received regional pain relief. It is also possible for an epidural/spinal itself to cause the baby's heart rate to slow (bradycardia), if, as noted above, the mother's blood pressure drops. Bradycardia can also occur after spinal narcotics are given. Your anesthesiologist is aware of these possibilities, and your baby's heart rate will be closely monitored. If it slows down, she or he will treat it by administering i.v. fluids and medications as needed.

RISK: INABILITY TO URINATE

Epidurals/spinals may numb the nerves of the bladder. If this happens, the laboring woman may not sense that her bladder is full. Sitting on the toilet, which is possible with a walking epidural, may enable her to urinate. In other cases, a urinary catheter may need to be inserted into her bladder to drain the urine. Studies show that compared to old-fashioned high-dose epidurals, low-dose epidurals or combined spinal-epidurals reduce the chance of not being able to urinate during labor. The baby's descent toward the birth canal sometimes blocks the flow of urine, so that insertion of a catheter into the bladder to drain the urine may be required even in women who don't have epidurals. Regardless of the type of epidural or spinal used, bladder sensation returns to normal as the anesthesia wears off.

RISK: PAIN DESPITE AN EPIDURAL/SPINAL

Sometimes women continue to feel labor pain even after receiving an epidural, for one of several reasons. First, the dose of pain medication may not have been strong enough. Each labor is different, which is why your anesthesiologist will individualize your treatment and give you just what you need— ideally, no more and no less. Here again, patient-controlled epidural analgesia (PCEA) makes this goal more achievable by allowing you to control the amount of pain relief you get.

Another reason you may still feel pain after receiving the epidural has to do with the position of your baby. If the baby descends into the birth canal face-up—that is, looking in the direction of the ceiling (known as the occiput posterior position)—labor tends to be more painful, especially in your lower back. Also, if the baby happens to be pressing directly on a nerve or nerves in your pelvis, it can be very painful, even with an epidural.

Another cause for pain despite having an epidural is rapid progression of your labor. For most women, the further labor advances, the more it hurts. If your labor is moving very quickly, the medication you initially received may not be enough to alleviate this more intense pain. In order to catch up with treating the increasing pain, you may need a booster dose of a stronger pain reliever—another reason it makes sense to get your epidural early. It is easier to get excellent control of the pain before it becomes severe, and then to add booster doses of stronger anesthetics as needed.

Sometimes, an epidural relieves pain on only one side the body. There is usually a straightforward explanation for this: the tip of the epidural catheter is located too far over to one side. When the catheter is inserted into your back, the chance of its staying exactly in the center of your epidural space is very small; it nearly always ends up on one side or the other. Although this usually is not a problem, if the catheter ends up too far to one side, it may not produce adequate pain relief on the other side. This situation can be corrected by pulling the catheter out a bit, a maneuver that tends to bring the tip closer to the center, producing equal pain relief on both sides of the body (figure 9-3).

Pregnant Pause

For one of several reasons, you may still feel pain even after you've had your epidural/spinal. If this happens, tell your anesthesiologist right away, so the necessary adjustments can be made to get you comfortable.

Another explanation for continued pain on only one side is gravity. For example, if you remain lying on your left side for a couple of hours, the medication tends to settle in the left side of your epidural space, causing you to feel pain only on your right side. This problem can be corrected, and prevented, by changing your position from your right to left side every so often.

If your epidural is working well but then stops working, the catheter may have become dislodged, so that the tip is no longer in the epidural space at all. This happens occasionally, and when it does, the catheter needs to be reinserted.

So if you experience pain despite having an epidural/spinal, be sure to tell your anesthesiologist right away. He or she can figure out the reason for it, and take some simple steps to remedy the situation so that you can labor in comfort.

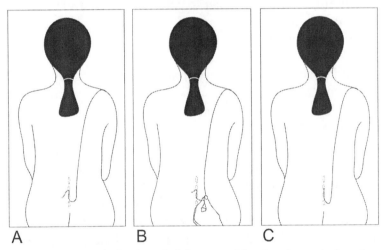

A   B   C

Fig. 9-3. *One-sided pain relief due to epidural catheter tip location. A: Catheter tip located too far to the woman's left side. B: Catheter being withdrawn slightly. C: Catheter tip now located in middle.*

EPIDURALS AND FEVER
Some laboring women who receive epidurals develop a higher temperature than those who do not. This is potentially problematic since maternal fever can alter the obstetrical management of labor and, for example, lead to a decision to perform a cesarean.

Also, an increase in maternal temperature is passively transmitted to the baby, and fever in the newborn may trigger tests to determine if an infection is present. And elevated temperatures may prompt physicians to administer antibiotics to mother and baby.

With regard to these issues—obstetrical intervention, testing of the newborn, and antibiotic administration—the entire clinical picture must be considered. If the mother's temperature does rise, it presents a challenge to physicians caring for her and her baby. This is where clinical judgment is important and the decision to alter labor management, to perform diagnostic tests, and to give antibiotics must be based on the entire clinical picture—not only on the mother's temperature. There are many harmless causes of a raised temperature; not every fever is due to an infection. Strenuous exercise, for example, can rapidly cause a fever.

More ominously, high fetal temperature has been associated with abnormal brain development and implicated in disorders such as cerebral palsy.[12] If epidurals do, in fact, cause maternal fevers, this could theoretically be harmful. But the relationship between epidurals and fevers is not fully understood. The key question is, are epidurals merely *associated* with fevers, or do they *cause* fevers?

Women with dysfunctional labor—labor that progress more slowly than normal—are more likely to develop fever because they undergo more vaginal exams, putting them at higher risk of developing inflammation of the membranes surrounding the baby (known as chorioamnionitis). Because these women are also more likely to receive epidurals, the epidurals may be wrongly blamed as the cause of the fevers. More research is needed to clarify this issue.

RARE RISKS OF EPIDURALS/SPINALS
The rare complications that may occur with epidurals and spinals can be classified into two categories: local and systemic.

Local complications refer to problems in the vicinity of the epidural/spinal spaces and include infection, bleeding, and nerve damage. Infection and bleeding are always possible when a needle is inserted anywhere in the body, and can potentially result in nerve damage or even paralysis if not diagnosed in time. Nerves may also be injured by the needle or catheter itself, or due to a reaction to the medication injected.

Systemic complications, which refer to problems that can affect your entire body, can occur if a high dose of anesthesia is unintentionally injected into the bloodstream, and include seizure or even death. Unintentional injection of a dose of anesthetic intended for the epidural space into the spinal space may cause slowing or stopping of breathing. Your anesthesiologist is trained to take every precaution to minimize the chance of these rare complications.

Just how rare are they? Because there is no database of all epidurals, spinals, and complications, we can only estimate their incidence from the scientific literature. The approximate chance of the type of infection known as an abscess caused by epidurals is estimated to be 1 in 150,000; bleeding in the epidural space, known as a hematoma, 1 in 170,000; spinal infection (meningitis) after the dura is punctured, 1 in 40,000; permanent nerve damage, 1 in 250,000; and the risk of temporary (reversible) nerve damage, 1 in 7,000. This last figure may be highly misleading, though, as most cases of temporary, reversible nerve damage are due to obstetric causes—that is, labor and delivery itself—and have nothing to do with the epidural or spinal.[13, 14]

Pregnant Pause

For some women, although the chance of a serious side effect is very small, the fear of a potential complication is enough to dissuade them from asking for an epidural or spinal. Ultimately, each person must make that decision for herself.

UNRELATED COMPLICATIONS

All sorts of troubles attributed to epidurals/spinals are not actually related. For example, a headache after delivery may have many causes, including lack of sleep or caffeine deprivation, or even an annoying roommate. If an epidural/spinal was given, however, all eyes are focused on the anesthesia, and nearly everyone concludes it must be a post-dural puncture headache.

Similarly, many causes of nerve injury during delivery have nothing to do with epidurals/spinals. A baby's head pressing on a nerve as it passes through the mother's pelvis can cause postpartum numbness and/or weakness. If forceps are used, they can irritate a nerve or two. But if the patient received an epidural/spinal, a convenient explanation is simply that the anesthesia must have caused the nerve injury. The good news is that although bothersome nerve symptoms may occur after childbirth whether or not an epidural/spinal is used, the symptoms typically improve gradually, with time.

PUTTING THE RISK IN PERSPECTIVE

It is important to keep the risks in perspective. Most likely, you've never had an epidural/spinal before, so it is understandable if you're concerned. In fact, it would be a little strange if you weren't. But it's important to remember that the overwhelming majority of women who receive epidurals/spinals for childbirth suffer no complications whatsoever. For the very few among whom complications occur, most experience only temporary difficulties. But some rare complications are associated with long-lasting problems; so although it's highly unlikely a serious complication will occur, it is important to understand the potential risks involved.

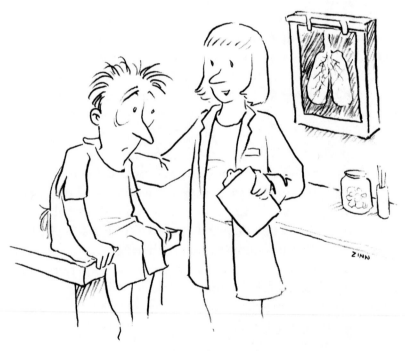

"Mr. Smith, all the tests show that you have pneumonia—so which will it be: penicillin or the natural approach?"

10

UNRELIEVED PAIN: THE RISKS OF NOT USING AN EPIDURAL OR SPINAL

Topics to Be Delivered

- **Harmful physiological effects of unrelieved pain for mother and baby**
- **How epidurals/spinals can prevent the physiological effects of pain**
- **Harmful psychological effects of unrelieved pain for mother and baby**
- **How epidurals/spinals may limit the psychological effects of pain**

When considering whether to use epidurals/spinals for childbirth, mothers-to-be and their obstetric caregivers review the potential risks—a sensible thing to do before any medical treatment or intervention. But they virtually never take into account the risks of *not* receiving regional pain relief. As recent studies have shown, these risks are quite real, and may result in serious complications.

PHYSIOLOGICAL EFFECTS OF CHILDBIRTH PAIN

Besides causing suffering, unrelieved pain carries potential harmful consequences for you and your baby. Most women hyperventilate during painful contractions—especially if labor breathing techniques are used improperly—and in addition to tingly hands, light-headedness, or even unconsciousness, hyperventilation can stop the normal impulse to breathe between contractions. That reduces oxygen in your blood, meaning less gets transferred through the placenta to your baby.

Pregnant Pause

Although most pregnant women are aware of at least some of the risks of getting an epidural or a spinal, few mothers-to-be ever consider the risks of *not* getting an epidural or spinal.

In addition, stressful situations like severe labor pain cause the body to release a lot of adrenaline into the bloodstream. Adrenaline narrows blood vessels throughout the body, including the blood vessels of the uterus that bring oxygen to the placenta. Therefore, when the mother experiences pain and stress, the baby receives less oxygen.

Epidurals/spinals stop the pain and thus reduce the adrenaline level in the blood. Although for most labors, constriction of blood vessels in response to pain does not make a difference, it is better for the baby to receive more than less oxygen. Labor is stressful enough for the baby as it is.

Pregnant Pause

Blood tests done at the time of birth show that babies of mothers who receive epidurals have a more favorable biochemical status than babies of mothers who do it naturally.

CONTROLLED PAIN, CONTROLLED DELIVERY

Epidural/spinal techniques let mothers be in control during the delivery. If you are in excruciating pain, it is much more difficult to comply with the instructions of your obstetrician or midwife. On the other hand, if you are comfortable, you can participate fully and assist your obstetrician or midwife to perform a controlled delivery. This in turn may reduce the trauma to your perineum.

A controlled delivery may also be better for your baby. This is especially true for premature babies, who are relatively more fragile than full-term babies and less able to tolerate forceful, rapid expulsion from the birth canal.

FROM BLUES TO DEPRESSION TO PTSD: POSTPARTUM EFFECTS OF UNTREATED PAIN

A few days after giving birth, some 50 to 80 percent of new mothers experience a condition commonly known as the "baby blues" or "postpartum blues," marked by mood swings, irritability, tearfulness, anxiety, insomnia, and fatigue. Because the blues occur in the majority of new moms, they are not considered pathological but rather a normal occurrence requiring no specific treatment, just support and encouragement.

Postpartum blues are typically short-lived, and usually gone by the time the newborn is ten days old. But if the blues continue for more than two weeks, it is possible a more serious problem has developed.

Postpartum depression, which occurs in approximately 10 to 15 percent of new mothers has been called "the thief that steals motherhood" by Cheryl Tatano Beck, a professor at the University of Connecticut School of Nursing who studies and writes extensively on the subject.[15] Unlike the limited-duration "blues," postpartum depression can last for months or longer and have devastating long-term effects on mother, baby and other family members.

Risk factors include a prior bout of depression after a previous delivery, a history of psychiatric illness—for example, depression unrelated to pregnancy—marital discord, extreme anxiety during pregnancy, stressful life events, and lack of social support from family and friends. And investigators have identified unrelieved pain during childbirth as an independent risk factor—for both postpartum depression and for post-traumatic stress disorder (PTSD).[16]

PTSD, a serious psychiatric illness that first gained widespread recognition among soldiers returning from the Vietnam War, can occur after experiencing or witnessing an extremely stressful situation involving actual or threatened death or serious injury to oneself or others. For women, a traumatic childbirth accompanied by fear, helplessness, loss of control, and pain can trigger PTSD.

In a 1998 study conducted in the U.K. at the University of Southampton School of Medicine, half the women who considered their labor to be traumatic perceived the pain as an indication that their life was being threatened.[17] While the incidence of full-blown PTSD after childbirth is 1 to 3 percent; the incidence of "partial" PTSD is likely much higher.[18]

As with postpartum depression, multiple factors can contribute to the development of PTSD, including pre-existing psychiatric disorders, negative experiences with a previous delivery, prior traumatic experiences, extreme anxiety, negative interactions with delivery staff, perceived inadequate care, lack of information and explanation, a low level of partner support, feelings of powerlessness, and fear for health of the baby, as may occur with an emergency cesarean delivery. Women with PTSD have nightmares and flashbacks of the experience, avoidance of things that may recall the experience—potentially even the baby—and other symptoms such as insomnia, anger, fear, hopelessness, inability to trust others, emotional detachment, sadness, lack of enjoyment, and loss of libido.

The repercussions can extend beyond the patient and the illness itself. A 2006 study conducted at the University of Heidelberg Medical School in Germany found that new mothers who were depressed during the first four months after delivery had lower-quality bonding with their infants during the first fourteen months of life.[19] Lack of adequate bonding during this critical period has been shown to result in impaired behavioral, emotional, interpersonal and possibly cognitive development through childhood.[15]

THE EFFECTS OF UNRELIEVED PAIN AFTER DELIVERY

A 2008 prospective study conducted jointly at Wake Forest and Columbia University Schools of Medicine found that pain after delivery may also predispose to postpartum depression.[20] Investigators found that women who experienced severe pain within thirty-six hours after delivery were three times more likely to develop postpartum depression than those who rated pain after delivery as mild. The incidence of postpartum depression was not related to whether the delivery was vaginal or cesarean; what mattered was the presence of severe pain itself.

Accumulating evidence shows that experiencing pain during and after surgery may predispose one to develop long-lasting pain—and it appears that childbirth pain is no exception. In the Wake Forest/Columbia study cited above, severe pain within thirty-six hours after childbirth—whether vaginal or cesarean—was associated with a 2.5 times greater chance of having persistent pain two months later. The investigators point out that providing optimal pain relief is especially important after childbirth, not only to limit the development of a chronic pain state but also to encourage healthy bonding between the new mother and her baby.[20] If the new mom is preoccupied dealing with her own pain, she will naturally be less inclined to interact as positively with her baby than if she were comfortable.

STIGMATIZATION

Women who suffer from postpartum depression or post-traumatic stress disorder are sometimes dismissed as weak or, worse, simply crazy. Needless to say, this type of societal response is not helpful for the woman in distress.

To counter this unfortunate situation, some women have organized to raise awareness of the problem, to give voice to those traumatized, and to advocate for better prevention and treatment. The Birth Trauma Association of the UK (www.birthtraumaassociation.org.uk) and Birth Trauma Canada (www.birthtraumacanada.org) are two such organizations.

Pregnant Pause

Research now suggests that pain experienced by the mother may contribute to the development of devastating psychiatric problems after delivery. So the pain of childbirth should not be regarded as causing only temporary suffering. Its effects may be long-lasting, and have serious consequences for the mother, her newborn, and her entire family.

PREVENTION OF POSTPARTUM PSYCHIATRIC CONDITIONS

Postpartum depression and post-traumatic stress disorder can be extremely difficult to treat. Experts therefore recommend identifying women at risk for developing these conditions long before their due date so that timely interventions can decrease the likelihood of their occurrence. During pregnancy, efforts can be made to reduce stress by having friends and family pitch in. The mother-to-be can be educated about the signs to be aware of after delivery. And if depression or PTSD does begin to develop, prompt treatment can be initiated.

Because the pain of childbirth has been identified as a risk factor for developing postpartum depression and PTSD, its elimination may reduce the chance that these illnesses will develop. In 1997 a Canadian Medical Association Journal article wisely stated that PTSD can and should be addressed by "providing excellent pain control during childbirth and careful postpartum care that includes understanding the woman's birth experience."[21]

Although pain is only one of many factors that can increase the chance of developing postpartum psychiatric illness, it is one we can completely control with epidurals/spinals—and especially with PCEA, which enables the woman to control and fine-tune her own pain relief throughout labor and delivery and during the immediate postpartum period. Everyone who plays a role in the field of obstetrics ought to consider that apart from its obvious immediate benefits, effective labor pain relief may also help prevent the development of long-lasting psychological trauma.

Key Concepts to Carry Away

Childbirth pain causes more than just suffering. It may also result in physiological side effects for mother and baby, including reductions in oxygen supply due to stress responses that can be prevented by epidurals/spinals. Unrelieved pain during labor and delivery and immediately thereafter is also associated with a greater chance of developing postpartum depression or post-traumatic stress disorder, as well as long-term pain. Before deciding whether you want an epidural/spinal for labor and delivery, you should also consider the risks of unrelieved pain itself.

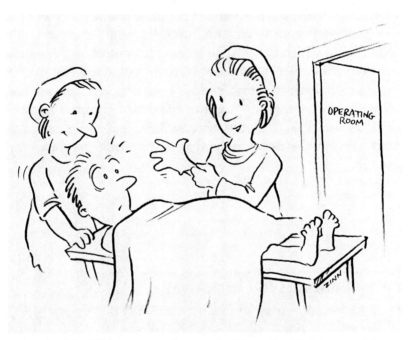

"Mr. Smith, I'll have your hemorrhoid out in 10 minutes. Were you thinking about getting anesthesia today, or did you want to do it naturally?"

11

CHILDBIRTH PAIN RELIEF: MYTHS AND REALITIES

 ### Topics to Be Delivered

- Do epidurals prolong labor?
- Is it a bad idea to get an epidural too early in labor?
- Will an epidural interfere with pushing?
- Is it ever too late to get an epidural?
- Do epidurals make it more likely that I will need a cesarean?
- Do epidurals make forceps or vacuum delivery more likely?
- If I move during the epidural placement will I become paralyzed?
- Will the epidural cause a long-lasting backache?
- Will the epidural interfere with breast-feeding?
- Can I get an epidural if I'm allergic to local anesthetics?
- If I have a slipped disc or if I have had back surgery, can I get an epidural?
- Will getting an epidural prevent me from eating or drinking during labor?
- Can I get an epidural if I have a low-back tattoo?

Many myths surround childbirth, and more than a few are related to pain relief techniques. Say something often enough, and people begin to believe it. The way to eradicate such untruths is through education. This chapter reviews commonly held misconceptions about epidurals/spinals along with the facts necessary to put them into perspective.

MYTH: IT'S A BAD IDEA TO GET AN EPIDURAL "TOO EARLY"

Reality: This corollary of the "epidural will slow down my labor" myth states that if you get epidural or spinal pain relief "too early," it will slow down labor and increase your chances of a forceps or cesarean delivery. This myth has been resoundingly debunked by four different prospective research studies of "early" epidurals/spinals published between 2005 and 2009. In these studies, women were divided into two groups: half the women had epidurals/spinals before four centimeters cervical dilation and half the women had epidurals/spinals after four centimeters dilation. In three of the studies, early administration of pain relief was associated with a quicker labor; in the fourth there was no difference in labor duration. Also, there was no difference in the likelihood of forceps or cesarean delivery in women who received the epidural/spinal early. Yet despite these data, this myth is still widespread among mothers-to-be and some obstetric caregivers.

Pregnant Pause

Although some people still adamantly believe that epidural pain relief slows the progress of labor, few would dispute that an epidural makes the experience a whole lot more comfortable.

MYTH: IF I HAVE AN EPIDURAL, I WON'T BE ABLE TO PUSH WELL

Reality: During the first stage of labor, uterine contractions dilate the cervix. During the second stage, you have a much more active role as you help to push the baby out. As mentioned above, the levels of medication traditionally used for epidurals prolonged the second stage an average of fifteen minutes, which is not the case with today's walking epidurals, so it all depends on the type of epidural that you have.

Beyond weakening of muscles, an epidural can conceivably prevent you from pushing effectively by blocking the pressure sensation as the baby descends. An epidural that is working very well may completely block the feeling of pressure normally sensed as the baby descends toward the birth canal. For most women, especially those delivering their first baby, this pressure serves as a focus for their pushing efforts. If the epidural eliminates the sensation entirely, pushing effectively may be more difficult, as was often the case with old-fashioned high-dose epidurals. Ideally, the epidural will relieve your pain but leave you with a feeling of pressure during the second stage.

The walking epidural minimizes muscle weakness—which, again, can prolong the second stage—while preserving the sensation of pressure by using very low doses of local anesthetics. Also, because the walking epidural affects pain nerves more than nerves that control muscle function, you retain the strength needed to push effectively. With patient-controlled epidural analgesia (PCEA), the mother-to-be can fine-tune the amount of pain relievers she receives, adjusting the intensity of pain relief to the point where the pain is blocked but muscle strength and the pressure sensation are maintained.

Pregnant Pause

An epidural does *not* have to be stopped during the pushing stage. Ideally, the pain-relieving medications are administered until the baby is born. With PCEA, you are able to fine-tune the amount of pain relief you receive, so that you can block the pain yet retain the sensation of pressure, which helps you to push more effectively.

MYTH: IT'S "TOO LATE" TO GET AN EPIDURAL

Reality: The "window of opportunity" misconception—that epidurals can't be given when the cervix is too far dilated—is the flip side of the too-early myth. Not only can an epidural be administered at any time once labor has been diagnosed or a decision to deliver the baby has been made, it can be given up to the very end of labor, when the cervix is completely dilated. This issue and controversies surrounding the timing of epidural and spinal pain relief are discussed fully in chapter 5.

MYTH: IF I GET AN EPIDURAL, I AM MORE LIKELY TO NEED A CESAREAN.

Reality: The myth that epidurals lead to an increased likelihood of cesarean still exists despite considerable evidence to the contrary. Although numbers alone may indicate an *association* between epidurals and cesarean delivery, closer examination of the data shows that epidurals do not *cause* cesareans. Since women who have difficult, prolonged labors and end up having a cesarean also tend to have more painful labors, they are likelier to request and receive epidurals—but their epidurals did not *cause* their cesareans. They would have needed a cesarean in any event. So one cannot simply compare epidural rates and cesarean rates and conclude that epidurals caused the cesareans.

"There's a problem with the way the literature has been interpreted," noted Dr. John Thorp, an obstetrician, in a 1997 *New York Times* article summarizing the roots of this myth. "There is a strong association between epidurals and cesareans, but not causality. Epidurals that were placed after an abnormal labor occurred can't be blamed for Cesareans."[23] Yet the myth persists.

MYTH: IF I GET AN EPIDURAL, I'M MORE LIKELY TO NEED A FORCEPS OR VACUUM DELIVERY

Reality: The data on this issue are not as clear-cut as they are for the epidural-cesarean issue, since not as much research has specifically addressed it. Forceps and vacuum deliveries do tend to occur more frequently in patients who receive epidurals. But, as with cesareans, the question is: are epidurals simply associated with forceps and vacuum deliveries, or do they cause them? Women with dysfunctional labors—that is, labors destined not to progress well, for whatever reason—are more likely to experience pain and to request an epidural. Women who have more intense labor pain are also likely to have a smaller chance of experiencing an easy vaginal delivery regardless of whether or not they received an epidural. The epidural given to relieve the pain is then blamed for the use of forceps or of a vacuum that may have ultimately been needed anyway. The question of causation with regard to epidurals and forceps/vacuum has not been completely resolved.

If the epidural prevents effective pushing, it stands to reason that epidurals would increase the rate of forceps and vacuum delivery. Since low-dose walking epidurals tend to preserve the ability to push, they should result in lower rates of forceps and vacuum deliveries. In fact, a study of 1,054 patients showed just that: low-dose epidural techniques resulted in a lower likelihood of the need for forceps and vacuum deliveries than did traditional higher-dose epidurals.[24] Clearly, low-dose walking epidurals—especially when combined with PCEA—are the way to go.

MYTH: IF I MOVE WHEN THE EPIDURAL NEEDLE IS BEING PLACED, I CAN BE PARALYZED

Reality: Your anesthesiologist understands it is difficult to remain completely still while you are feeling an excruciating contraction. In fact, you are expected to move during severe labor pain; most of my patients are moving around quite a bit when I insert their epidural. But that does not correlate with becoming paralyzed. In reality, if you were to suddenly move during the procedure, the worst result would likely be a spinal headache if the needle were to make a hole in the dura (chapter 9). Unfortunately, this myth commonly causes unnecessary worry in women considering an epidural/spinal.

MYTH: IF I HAVE AN EPIDURAL, I WILL END UP WITH A BACKACHE

Reality: Many women suffer backache during pregnancy as the weight of the baby increases stress on the muscles and ligaments of the spine. Women fortunate enough to get through pregnancy without backache may see one develop during labor and delivery. And backache after delivery is also common, lasting for days, weeks or even months. Not surprisingly, some women who have an epidural blame the pain relief technique for their backache: "I was fine before I had that needle in my back." But scientific investigation of this issue has clearly shown that epidurals do not cause backaches. We now know that the chance of developing a long-lasting backache after giving birth is identical whether or not an epidural is used.

Pregnant Pause
Although the scientific evidence shows that epidurals do not cause backaches, many people continue to believe that they do—a classic example of "don't confuse the argument with facts."

MYTH: IF I GET AN EPIDURAL, IT WILL INTERFERE WITH BREAST-FEEDING

Reality: While it has not been proved that epidurals interfere with breast-feeding the infant, some breast-feeding proponents argue this point passionately. They believe that the walking epidurals' low dose of synthetic narcotic (e.g., fentanyl, sufentanil) may have an adverse effect on the newborn, compromising its ability to breast-feed. And a study published in 2005 seemed to confirm their concerns, finding that breast-feeding rates at six weeks after delivery were lower in mothers who had received a higher dose of epidural narcotic during labor.[25] Yet the investigators found no significant effect on breast-feeding success on the day after delivery. There is no obvious scientific explanation for this finding: that a relatively small dose of short-acting narcotic administered to a woman during labor has no effect on breast-feeding success the day after delivery, but does have an effect six weeks later. The research has also been criticized for potentially serious flaws in study design.[26] Nonetheless, some staunch breast-feeding advocates have latched onto its conclusions, so to speak.

Another study published in 2010 assessed the influence of low-dose epidural narcotic during labor on subsequent nursing. The authors found that the use of epidural narcotic had no negative effect on breast-feeding.[27]

Successful breast-feeding depends on many factors, including the mother's motivation and the support she receives. To date, the science does not permit us to conclude that modern low-dose walking epidurals/spinals have a negative influence on breast-feeding success. More studies of this issue are needed.

Contrast this with the effects that systemic pain relievers taken by the mother have on the baby. Morphine or Demerol makes the mother sleepy, and the breast-feeding baby becomes sleepy as well. This is much less likely with an epidural, where the amount of medication that enters the bloodstream is quite small or with a spinal, where the amount is even smaller. And again, as mentioned in chapter 8, if a woman has suffered from severe after-pains while breast-feeding in the past, she may be reluctant to even attempt it this time around. For these women, leaving the epidural in place to provide pain relief after delivery may actually promote breast-feeding. Human behavior is adversely affected by pain. Suffering in pain exhausts a considerable amount of our energies. It stands to reason that a new mother experiencing pain from whatever cause, e.g., from vaginal birth-related perineal injury or from her cesarean incision, would be less attentive to breast-feeding her newborn—yet another reason to strive for a painless post-partum experience.

MYTH: NO PAIN, NO GAIN

Reality: While this approach may or may not be true for an exercise program, it is patently false for labor. Can you imagine that argument being made to a man about to undergo "minor" surgery for hemorrhoids? In a 1999 *New York Times Magazine* article, Margaret Talbot, who underwent both a "natural" and an epidural labor experience, wrote that "today's natural-child-birth purists ... regard labor as an extreme sport—an ennobling physical challenge that we pampered First Worlders are supposed to courageously endure and savor. Spurning the palliatives of modern medicine is part of the drill, an emblem of virtue. ...Yet what matters, surely, is not how you get through labor but that you get through it."[28]

MYTH: I HAVE AN ALLERGY TO LOCAL ANESTHETICS, SO I CAN'T GET AN EPIDURAL

Reality: True allergy to a local anesthetic is rare. Most of the time, women relate a story in which they have had some type of bad reaction to a local anesthetic at the dentist's office. In many cases, the perceived "allergy" may be explained by a small amount of adrenaline, which is often added to the local anesthetic, being injected into a blood vessel. This typically causes very unpleasant symptoms including trembling and a feeling that your heart is racing. But it is unlikely the reaction was caused by a true allergy to the local anesthetic.

The other main component of regional pain relief is a synthetic narcotic. Allergies to synthetic narcotics are also rare, and again highly unlikely. Before you go into labor it is possible to be tested to see if you have true allergies to any pain reliever you may receive, although the tests themselves are not 100 percent accurate. If you are concerned about a potential allergy to a pain reliever, you should discuss it with an anesthesiologist long in advance of your due date, so that a plan can be devised.

MYTH: I CAN'T HAVE AN EPIDURAL BECAUSE I HAVE A HERNIATED DISC

Reality: Having a herniated or bulging disc does not mean you can't get an epidural. In fact, many people who have pain caused by herniated discs are actually treated with epidural injections. A common misconception is that if there is already a problem in the lower back, why chance worsening it by putting a needle there? In fact, the discs between your vertebrae are located on the front side of the dura. Because an epidural is performed from behind the spine, the needle does not even get near the disc (figures 3-1 and 3-2).

Some anesthesiologists avoid using an epidural in a woman with a disc problem for fear the epidural will be blamed if symptoms happen to worsen afterward. Fact is, delivery itself may worsen the symptoms of a herniated or bulging disc whether or not an epidural is used. So the good news is that if you have a disc problem and you want an epidural, it's no problem. Other back problems such as scoliosis should not prevent you from getting an epidural either. In fact, many women who have undergone major back surgery have received epidurals for labor pain relief.

MYTH: I CAN'T EAT OR DRINK ONCE I HAVE THE EPIDURAL

Reality: In most hospitals in the United States, having the epidural does not limit your right to eat or drink, but being in labor does. Since the course and outcome of labor are not predictable, and there is a chance you may require general anesthesia for an emergency cesarean, it is best that your stomach be relatively empty to avoid aspiration, the spilling of stomach contents into the lungs. So once you're in labor, the policy at most hospitals nationwide is that you cannot have any solid foods, aspiration of which is more damaging than liquids. This is also the position of the American College of Obstetricians and Gynecologists and of the American Society of Anesthesiologists. The old-fashioned approach was to avoid liquids as well, but the thinking on this one has changed. It's certainly much more pleasant if you can have something to drink if you're thirsty. Nowadays, it's generally acceptable that a woman in labor be allowed to drink moderate amounts of clear liquids, that is, liquids that don't contain solid particles—whether or not she has an epidural.

Interestingly, in Great Britain, the attitude is much more permissive. There, women are routinely allowed to eat solid food during labor, and the data from the last twenty-five years show it seems to be safe for the mother. So, who knows? Maybe we'll loosen our rules for eating during labor on this side of the pond too. But don't plan to order in a gourmet meal just yet.

MYTH: I CAN'T HAVE AN EPIDURAL IF I HAVE A TATTOO OVER MY LOWER BACK

Reality: Having a tattoo on your back has nothing to do with getting an epidural. This myth had its origins a few years ago, when a report was published of one woman who had a labor epidural placed through a tattoo on her lower back. Afterward, she had some tenderness and burning at the site of the epidural. Although her symptoms resolved in less than twenty-four hours, some folks thought her symptoms may have been caused by the needle passing through the tattoo. No scientific data support this view, and countless other women with extensive tattoos have received epidurals without incident. Also, it's not uncommon for an epidural to cause some tenderness in the area for a day or two afterward, much like a "bruise" feeling. So tattoos really don't present a problem at all. If you have a one on your lower back, and you want an epidural, don't give this myth another thought.

Key Concepts to Carry Away

Misconceptions abound about epidural/spinal pain relief. Be sure you know the difference between myth and reality when choosing which, if any, pain relief you want for childbirth.

12

TIME FOR SOME NEW THINKING

Topics to Be Delivered

- **Epidurals and spinals do more than relieve temporary pain and suffering**
- **Is it really worth chancing a painful, stressful childbirth?**

It has been more than 160 years since the first woman received "modern" anesthesia for childbirth. Since then, the science and technology for providing pain relief for women in labor has evolved considerably. Mothers are no longer rendered unconscious for delivery. And unlike their forebears, women today can choose to experience childbirth in comfort. With epidurals/spinals, the pain of childbirth can be completely eliminated without causing drowsiness. The Lamaze movement that became popular in the 1960s has largely been eclipsed by an embrace of medical progress. In the United States today, more than 70 percent of women receive epidural/spinal pain relief during labor and delivery. Some mothers-to-be make a fully informed choice to forgo epidural/spinal pain relief. But others are dissuaded from choosing these techniques because of persistent myths and misconceptions.

CHANGE IS DIFFICULT

Old ideas die hard. Long after forward-thinkers had proved the earth was round, flat earth societies continued to flourish. Although the science of pain relief for childbirth now enables women to safely deliver in comfort, some don't take advantage of the option. Others call it "unnatural" interference in the way things are supposed to be. Even today, in the twenty-first century, there are those who believe women are meant to experience pain during labor and delivery. They assert that not experiencing the pain deprives a mother of the full measure of her womanhood, while somehow diminishing her worth. So, many women still continue to suffer through the experience of childbirth, primarily out of fear, guilt, and lack of accurate information.

LUXURY OR NECESSITY?

Even the fiercest critics of regional pain relief acknowledge that epidurals/spinals do a better job of relieving childbirth pain than any other method. But epidurals/spinals may do a lot more than just relieve the pain and suffering of the moment. As we have seen, accumulating evidence suggests that traumatic birth experiences may result in psychiatric illnesses like postpartum depression and post-traumatic stress disorder (PTSD), whose repercussions can cause long-term difficulties for mother, baby, and other family members. Evidence also indicates that pain *after* delivery can adversely affect the new mother's mental health, and that pain of vaginal and cesarean delivery may increase the chance of developing a chronic pain condition. If a woman chooses not to use an epidural/spinal, shouldn't she at least understand the potential consequences of that decision?

I maintain that in view of the accumulating evidence regarding the potential of pain relief to benefit the mother and baby not only during labor and delivery but also beyond, it is time for a complete rethink on the subject. Perhaps instead of asking, "Will I want an epidural for my delivery?" the question should be, "Do I really want to take the chance of depriving myself of state-of-the-art pain relief during my labor, delivery, and the immediate postpartum period?"

I do not mean to suggest that eliminating pain categorically prevents the occurrence of postpartum depression or PTSD. It is clear that many factors contribute to the development of these postpartum psychiatric conditions. But if pain is one factor you can control, doesn't it make sense to minimize it?

Once you arrive in the labor and delivery suite, your obstetrician, midwife, nurse, or doula should advocate for you to receive the best possible pain relief, and to give you the information you need to be in as much control of your situation as possible. Patient-controlled epidural analgesia, in which you can fine-tune the amount of pain-relieving medication you receive, is one way to be in more control. Knowing all of your options and understanding the risks and benefits of each is another. And being treated courteously and with dignity by the staff and being informed every step of the way is a prerequisite as much as a right.

Although all procedures involve risk, for the overwhelming majority of women, epidurals/spinals cause no serious complications. Given what I know about their advantages and disadvantages, I conclude it is riskier not to use epidurals/spinals than to use them. Of course, my conclusion doesn't really matter much to you; you are the one who has to make this decision for yourself. Only your decision matters.

I realize that my way of thinking represents a radical departure from the way people have thought about epidurals/spinals until now. And I can already hear the naysayers, those who will claim I am trying to frighten women into using epidurals/spinals. But we must adapt to new findings; that's what medicine has always been about. We are constantly evolving, constantly changing treatment as our understanding advances. If we are not open to change, we will never progress.

My goal in writing *Epidural Without Guilt* has been to bring the facts about modern pain relief for childbirth to light, and to demystify the techniques in use today, so you can decide whether to take advantage of these medical miracles during your delivery. I sincerely hope that in so doing, I have addressed your concerns. I believe that understanding your options is empowering. If I have encouraged you to seek further information and to consult with your obstetrician or midwife and anesthesiologist well in advance of your labor, then I have succeeded in my task. Ultimately, it is your right—and yours alone—to decide what type of pain relief, if any, you would like to receive. But if you choose an epidural/spinal, do it without guilt, and with full knowledge of the benefits and risks involved. It's your body and it's your decision.

Key Concepts to Carry Away

While they're already acknowledged to be the most effective way to relieve the pain of childbirth, new data suggest epidurals/spinals may have another important role. By stopping pain, they may help prevent devastating psychiatric illness in the new mother, such as postpartum depression and post-traumatic stress disorder. The appropriate question for today is: Should anyone giving birth be deprived of this advantage?

NOTES

1. Kathleen Berrin and Thomas K Seligman, *Art of the Huichol Indians* (New York: Harry N. Abrams, 1978), 162.

2. Peter Brownridge, "The nature and consequences of childbirth pain," *European Journal of Obstetrics & Gynecology and Reproductive Biology* 59 Suppl., 1995. S9-15.

3. Edward Wagenknecht, *Mrs. Longfellow: Selected Letters and Journals of Fanny Appleton Longfellow (1817-1861)* (New York: Longmire Green & Co., 1956), 129-130.

4. Donald Caton, *What a Blessing She Had Chloroform: The Medical and Social Response to the Pain of Childbirth from 1800 to the Present* (New Haven: Yale University Press, 1999), 20-53, 90-129.

5. Angel Vahratian, et al., "The effect of early epidural versus early intravenous analgesia use on labor progression: A natural experiment," *American Journal of Obstetrics and Gynecology* 191, no. 1, July 2004. 259-265.

6. Cynthia A. Wong, et al., "The risk of cesarean delivery with neuraxial analgesia given early versus late in labor," *New England Journal of Medicine* 352, no. 7, February 2005. 655-665.

7. Cynthia A. Wong, et al., "Early compared with late neuraxial analgesia in nulliparous labor induction: A randomized controlled trial," *Obstetrics and Gynecology* 113, no. 5, May 2009. 1066-1074.

8. Gonen Ohel et al., "Early versus late initiation of epidural analgesia in labor: Does it increase the risk of cesarean section? A randomized trial," *American Journal of Obstetrics and Gynecology* 194, no. 3. March 2006. 600-605.

9. FuZhou Wang et al., "Epidural analgesia in the latent phase of labor and the risk of cesarean delivery: A five-year randomized controlled trial," *Anesthesiology* 111, no. 4, October 2009. 871-880.

10. Michael Wuitchik, Donald Bakal, and Jeffrey Lipshitz, "The clinical significance of pain and cognitive activity in latent labor," *Obstetrics and Gynecology* 73, no. 1, January 1989. 35-42.

11. American College of Obstetricians and Gynecologists, "ACOG Committee Opinion No. 339: Analgesia and cesarean delivery rates," *Obstetrics and Gynecology* 107, June 2006. 1487-1488.

12. Joy L. Hawkins, "Epidural analgesia for labor and delivery," *New England Journal of Medicine* 362, no. 16, April 2010. 1503-1510.

13. Felicity Reynolds, "Neurological infections after neuraxial anesthesia," *Anesthesiology Clinics* 26, no. 1, March 2008. 23-52.

14. Wilhelm Ruppen et al., "Incidence of epidural hematoma, infection, and neurologic injury in obstetric patients with epidural analgesia/anesthesia," *Anesthesiology* 105, no. 2, August 2006. 394-399.

15. Cheryl Tatano Beck, "Postpartum depression: It isn't just the blues," *American Journal of Nursing* 106, no. 5, May 2006. 40-50.

16. Pauliina Hiltunen et al., "Does pain relief during delivery decrease the risk of postnatal depression?" *Acta Obstetrica and Gynecologica Scandinavica* 83, no. 3, March 2004. 257-261.

17. Sarah Allen, "A qualitative analysis of the process, mediating variables and impact of traumatic childbirth," *Journal of Reproductive and Infant Psychology* 16, no. 2 & 3, May 1998. 107-131.

18. Kristie Alcorn et al., A prospective longitudinal study of the prevalence of posttraumatic stress disorder resulting from childbirth events," *Psychological Medicine* 40, no.11, November 2010. 1849-59.

19. Eva Moehler et al., "Maternal depressive symptoms in the postnatal period are associated with long-term impairment of mother-child bonding," *Archives of Women's Mental Health* 9, no. 5, September 2006. 273-8.

20. James C. Eisenach, "Severity of acute pain after childbirth, but not type of delivery, predicts persistent pain and postpartum depression," *Pain* 140, no. 1, September 2008. 87-94.

21. J. Lawrence Reynolds, "Post-traumatic stress disorder after childbirth: The phenomenon of traumatic birth," *Canadian Medical Association Journal* 156, no. 6. March 1997. 831-835.

22. Steven H. Halpern and Barbara L. Leighton, "Misconceptions about neuraxialanalgesia," *Anesthesiology Clinics of North America* 21. 2003. 59-70.

23. Susan Gilbert, "No cesarean risk is found for a labor pain medication," *New York Times*. October 21, 1997. F9.

24. Comparative Obstetric Mobile Epidural Trial (COMET) Study Group UK. "Effect of low-dose mobile versus traditional epidural techniques on mode of delivery: A randomised controlled trial," *Lancet* 358, no. 9275, July 2001. 19-23.

25. Yaakov Beilin et al., "Effect of labor epidural analgesia with and without fentanyl on infant breast-feeding; a prospective, randomized, double-blind study," *Anesthesiology* 103, no. 6, December 2005. 1211-1217.

26. Steven H. Halpern and Alexander Ioscovich. Epidural analgesia and breast-feeding. *Anesthesiology* 103, no. 6, December 2005. 1111-1112.

27. Paul M. Wieczorek, "Breastfeeding success rate after vaginal delivery can be high despite the use of epidural fentanyl: an observational cohort study," *International Journal of Obstetric Anesthesia* 19, no. 3. July 2010. 273-277.

28. Margaret Talbot, "Pay on Delivery," *New York Times Magazine*, Oct. 31, 1999. 19-20.

GLOSSARY

ACOG – American College of Obstetricians and Gynecologists. It has over 46,000 members and is the nation's leading group of professionals providing health care for women.

Adrenaline (epinephrine) – A chemical produced in the adrenal glands, especially during times of stress. Among other effects, adrenaline narrows blood vessels, including those of the uterus, thus reducing the amount of oxygen that is brought to the baby.

After-pains – Abdominal pains due to contractions of the uterus after the baby is born, which are worsened by breast-feeding; they tend to increase in severity with each successive birth.

Analgesia – The relief of pain without the loss of consciousness.

Anesthesia – The loss of pain sensation as in surgery, with or without the loss of consciousness.

APGAR – A scoring system to rate the well-being of a baby during the first few minutes of life; devised by American anesthesiologist Virginia Apgar.

Aspiration – The spilling of stomach contents into the lungs as may occur in an unconscious person.

Asphyxia – the condition in which there is a lack of oxygen and a buildup of carbon dioxide leading to loss of consciousness or death.

Birth canal – The lower portion of the uterus, the cervix and the vagina through which the baby passes during delivery.

Bonding – The process in which a close, loving relationship develops between the baby and the parents after birth.

Bradycardia – Slow heart rate.

Breech – The baby's position in the uterus where the feet or buttocks are poised to emerge first, before the head.

Cervix – The opening at the outlet of the uterus through which the baby passes during the delivery.

Chorioamnionitis – inflammation of membranes that surround the baby due to a bacterial infection.

Combined spinal-epidural (CSE) – A regional pain relief technique in which both a spinal and an epidural are performed at the same time.

Dilate, dilation – The widening of a structure to a larger size.

Dura – A layer of tissue that covers the brain and spinal cord, and surrounds the spinal fluid.

EKG (electrocardiogram) – A recording of the electrical activity of the heart; used to monitor heart function.

Electronic infusion pump – A device that can be programmed to give a specific dose of medication. It may be used to provide a steady dose and/or to give intermittent doses in response to patient need. See patient controlled analgesia (PCA) and patient controlled epidural analgesia (PCEA).

Epidural – A space within the vertebral column, outside the dura, through which nerves travel. Also, the anesthetic technique in which medication is injected to block the pain signal from traveling through the nerves, to keep the patient pain-freeand awake.

Epidural blood patch – A procedure to treat post-spinal headaches, in which approximately one-half ounce of the patient's blood is taken from a forearm vein, and is injected into the epidural space. The blood forms a clot that seals the hole in the dura, which prevents the further leakage of spinal fluid. See also Spinal headache.

Epidural catheter – A tiny soft, flexible plastic tube through which pain relieving medications are injected into the epidural space.

Epidural needle – A specially designed needle that is placed into the epidural space in order to inject medications and/or fluids, and through which an epidural catheter may be passed.

Epinephrine – See Adrenaline.

Episiotomy – A controlled surgical incision of the perineum performed by the obstetrician to limit the tearing of tissues during the delivery of the baby.

First stage of labor – See stages of labor.

Forceps – Instruments sometimes used by the obstetrician to help deliver the baby.

Hyperventilation – Rapid breathing

Intravenous (i.v.) – Literally "in the vein," it refers to the needle or small plastic tube that is placed into a vein to administer fluids and/or medications.

i.v. – See Intravenous

Intubation – The act of inserting a plastic tube into the trachea (windpipe) in order to administer oxygen and anesthetic gases.

Midazolam (Versed) – A medication related to Valium that may be given through the i.v., which produces sedation and relieves anxiety.

Obstetric anesthesiologist – An anesthesiologist who provides pain relief for labor and delivery, and in the postpartum period.

Occiput posterior – the position in which the baby's head is delivered facing toward the ceiling; may be associated with more painful labor, especially in the lower back.

Oxytocin – See Pitocin.

Patient controlled analgesia (PCA) – A technique in which the patient controls her own dosing of pain relievers that are injected into her i.v. by pushing a button connected to an electronic infusion pump. The pump is programmed to prevent overdosing.

Patient controlled epidural analgesia (PCEA) – A technique in which the patient controls her own dosing of pain relievers that are injected into her epidural catheter by pushing a button connected to an electronic infusion pump. The pump is programmed to prevent overdosing.

Perineum (perineal area) – The region between the vagina and the anus.

Pitocin – A synthetic form of the hormone oxytocin; given by the obstetrician to cause uterine contractions.

Post-dural puncture headache – See spinal headache.

Post partum – The interval after the delivery of the baby.

Pulse oximeter – A small device that is placed on a finger to measure the amount of oxygen in the blood.

Regional pain relief – The technique of administering pain relieving medication to eliminate pain in a specific area (region)of the body; for example, epidurals and spinals.

Resuscitation – Restoring breathing and blood circulation to a patient in distress.

Second stage of labor – See stages of labor.

Spinal – The term used to describe pain relief that is achieved by injecting medication into the cerebrospinal fluid.

Spinal cord – The cluster of nerves located within the vertebral column through which signals are transmitted from the body to the brain.

Spinal fluid – The fluid surrounding and cushioning the brain and spinal cord.

Spinal headache – Also called post-dural puncture headache. It results from the leakage of cerebrospinal fluid through a hole in the dura created by a spinal or epidural needle.

Spinous processes – The parts of the spinal bones that can be felt as small bumps along the center of the back. The anesthesiologist feels these bumps in order to determine precisely where to place the epidural or spinal needle.

Stages of labor –
   First Stage – The portion of labor from the onset of regular contractions, which cause the cervix to change shape, until full dilation of the cervix (ten centimeters) is reached.
   Second Stage – The portion of labor from full dilation of the cervix until the delivery of the baby.
   Third Stage – The interval from the birth of the baby to the delivery of the placenta.

Stat – Immediately

Synthetic narcotic – A man-made pain reliever similar in chemical structure and function to morphine.

Systemic pain relief – The technique in which pain relieving medication is administered into a vein, a muscle or taken by mouth, and is then distributed throughout the entire body(system).

Trachea (windpipe) – The tubular structure in the neck through which air from the mouth and nose travels to the lungs.

Third stage of labor – See stages of labor.

Uterus – The womb; the pelvic organ in which the baby grows.

Vacuum delivery – application of suction via a (plastic) cup placed on the baby's head to help guide the baby out of the birth canal.

Versed – see Midazolam.

Walking epidural – A technique in which a low-dose of a local anesthetic, usually combined with a synthetic narcotic, is given to produce pain relief with a minimum of muscle weakness, to enable the mother to walk if she desires, and to push effectively during the second stage of labor.

INDEX

ACOG (American College of Obstetrics and Gynecology): position on epidurals, 43
adrenaline and stress, 86
after-pains, 63-65
allergic reaction to epidural, 100
anesthesia, general: and aspiration, 54; and cesarean, 53–56; and preparation for, 58; and unanticipated situations, 57.
anesthesiologist: and administration of epi-dural/spinal, 47-51; availability of during labor, 44; and drop in patient's blood pressure, 58-59, 76; and explanation of procedures to patient, 50; and prevention of complications, 82; and systemic pain relief, 13-14; training of, 28
anxiety, 1
Apgar score and risk of systemic narcotics, 21
aorta, and low blood pressure, 77
aspiration, 54

baby's heart rate. See bradycardia
backache, and epidural, 98
"back labor," 13
bed rest, and spinal headache, 74-75
bleeding. *See* rare risks of epidurals and spinals
blood clotting disorder, 55-56
blood pressure. *See* decreased blood pressure, low blood pressure
blood pressure cuff, 48, 58

blues, postpartum, 87
booster doses, 34. *See also* PCEA
bradycardia (slowing of baby's heart rate), 78; and cesarean, 54
breast engorgement, 72
breast-feeding: and after-pains, 63-64; and epidural, 98-99
breathing tube, 54
Brownridge, Dr. Peter, 10
butorphanol. *See* Stadol

catheter, urinary 78
Caton, Dr. Donald: *What a Blessing She Had Chloroform: The Medical and Surgical Response to the Pain of Childbirth from 1800 to the Present,* 18
"caudal" procedure, 22
cervix: dilation of, 12, 32, 37–38; and dysfunctional labor, 41-42; and timing of epidural, 38-41, 94, 95
cesarean, 32, 41, 53-61, 66; and blood pressure, 76; and causing of, with epidural, 96; and general vs. regional anesthesia, 54–56; and epidural and spinal narcotics after, 68; and mobility, 68; and PCA, 68; and PCEA, 65; and perception of failure, 61; and postoperative pain, 65; and timing of epidural, 38-41
cesarean, stat (emergency), 53
Channing, Dr. Walter, 19
childbirth education classes, 1
childbirth, natural. See natural childbirth

childbirth pain: and double standard, 5; and Huichol Indians, 6-7; and prejudice, 6

childbirth pain relief: and ether, 18; and feelings of guilt, 9; history of, 17–28; natural or unnatural, 7–8; and opposition to, 18-19; perceptions of, 5–10;

chloroform, 18, 19

climax, and Orgasmic Birth, 6

combined spinal-epidural, 27, 28 (figure 3-7), 31, 32, 33, 57

complications, of epidurals and spinals, 71-83

contractions: after delivery, 63-64, 83; compared to menstrual cramps, 12; and intravenous fluids, 76-77; and systemic narcotics, 13-14

controlled delivery, 87

data about early epidurals, 38-41

decreased blood pressure, 76-77; effect of mother's position on, 77; and regional anesthetics, 76-77; and slowing of baby's heart rate, 78. *See also* low blood pressure

delivery, and epidural, 94-95

Demerol (meperidine), 13, 20; and breast-feeding newborns, 99; risks of, to baby, 20

depression, postpartum, 87; effect on bonding, 89; implications childhood development, 89; incidence with severe postpartum pain, 89; prevention of, 90-91, 104-105, 106; risk factors for, 88

double standard, 5-6

dura, 22, (figure 3-1), 25, 26; puncturing of, and treatment, 75–76 (figure 9-2). *See also* spinal headache

Duramorph (morphine), after cesarean, 67

dysfunctional labor, 41-42

eating and drinking with epidural, 101-102

effects of systemic pain medication on baby, 20-21, 65

effects of general anesthesia on baby, 18, 54

EKG (electrocardiogram), 48, 58

electronic pump, 25, 33–35, 43-44, 66-67. *See also* epidural catheter, epidural infusion pump

epidural, 13-15; advantages of, 14, 15; and cesarean delivery myth, 96; combined with spinal, 27-28 (figure 3-7), 31–33; at early stage of labor, 37-38; length of time to relieve pain, 31, 42; procedure, 22–24 (figures 3-2, 3-3), 48-51 (figures 6-1, 6-2); technological advances of, 25–26; timing of, during labor, 31-32, 37–46. *See also* combined epidural-spinal, epidural myths, PCA, PCEA, spinal, walking epidural

epidural blood patch, 75-76 (figure 9-2). See also spinal headache

epidural catheter, 23-24 (figures 3-3, 3-4, 3-7); 23, 24, 44, 47; description of, 50-51; in early labor, 43; and emergency cesarean, 54-56; and pain with position of, 79-80

after vaginal delivery, 63-65, 68-69; and unrelieved pain, 85-91; and uterine contractions, 78-79

postpartum numbness, 83

postpartum psychological trauma, 87-91, 104-106

postpartum weakness, 83

post-traumatic stress disorder (PTSD), 88; causes of, 88; effect on bonding, 89; incidence with severe postpartum pain, 89; prevention of, 90-91, 104-105, 106; risk factors for, 88; triggered by traumatic childbirth, 88

premature baby and controlled delivery, 87

pressure sensation, 95

pushing stage of labor, 12

Queen Victoria, 18

quickly moving labor, 79

rare risks of epidurals and spinals, 81-82

Regional pain relief: definition of, 13-15, 21-22; advantages of, 13-15; and decreased blood pressure, 76-77; and inability to urinate, 78; risks of, 71-84; reasons for not using, 54-56; and spinal headache, 26, 72-76; types of regional anesthesia, 21-24. *See also* risks of not using an epidural or spinal

resuscitation, 28

risks of not using an epidural or spinal and unrelieved pain,

85-91; adrenaline and stress, 86; avoidance of general anesthesia, 57; effect on nursing baby, 98-99; pain and postpartum depression, 87-91, 104, 106

saddle block, 42

second stage of labor, 32; and pain relief, 44

Simpson, Dr. James Young, 18

skin infection and risks, 55

sleep deprivation, and headache, 83

sleep during labor, 30

slowing down labor, and epidural, 94

Snow, Dr. John, 18

spinal, 26-27, 47–52; anticipation of, 47; and baby's heart rate, 78; and cesarean, 57; combined with epidural, 27, 28 (figure 3-7), 31–33, 51-53; disadvantages of, 26; length of time to relieve pain, 26; in late labor, 32; request for, in labor, 42; risks of, 71-83. *See also* epidural, combined epidural-spinal

spinal cord, 22 (figure 3-1)

spinal disc, 22 (figure 3-1)

spinal fluid, 22 (figure 3-1), 51; leakage of, 73-74. *See also* spinal headache

spinal headache, 72-75, incidence of, 73; left untreated, 74; position of body with, 74; treatment of, 75-76

spinal needle. *See* pencil point needle

spouse (or partner) at cesarean

ABOUT THE AUTHOR

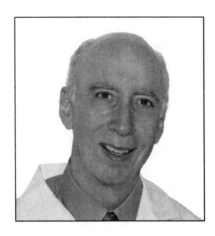

Dr. Gilbert J. Grant earned his BA at the University of Michigan in 1978 and his medical degree from the University of Michigan Medical School in 1982. After completing an internship in obstetrics and gynecology at Columbia Presbyterian Hospital in New York and a residency in anesthesiology at New York University Medical Center, in 1986 Dr. Grant joined the Department of Anesthesiology of New York University Medical Center, where he is currently an associate professor, the director of obstetric anesthesia, and a vice chairman for academic affairs.

In addition to his medical practice, Dr. Grant has continuously been engaged in clinical and laboratory research focused on improving patient care. He was an active participant in the changeover from the "old-fashioned" epidural in vogue at the beginning of his career to the "walking" epidural he now routinely administers. Since 1989 he has worked on developing an ultra-long-acting local anesthetic designed to provide sustained pain relief. Dr. Grant has published numerous scientific papers and chapters for medical textbooks, and he lectures at educational institutions and scientific meetings in the United States and abroad.

Proprietary pharmaceuticals mentioned in this book:

Trade Name	Generic Name	Manufacturer
Demerol	meperidine	Sanofi-Aventis US, LLC
Duramorph	preservative-free morphine	ESI Lederle Generics
Motrin	ibuprofen	McNeil Consumer Healthcare
Narcan	naloxone	Endo Laboratories, LLC
Nubain	nalbuphine	Endo Laboratories, LLC
Pitocin	oxytocin	Pfizer US Pharmaceuticals Group
Stadol	butorphanol	Bristol-Myers Squibb
Tylenol	acetaminophen	Johnson & Johnson/ Merck Consumer
Valium	diazepam	Roche Pharmaceuticals
Versed	midazolam	Roche Pharmaceuticals

CPSIA information can be obtained at www.ICGtesting.com
227852LV00008B/55/P